C000140108

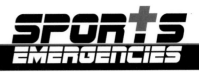

SPORTS
EMERGENCIES

Commissioning Editors: Claire Wilson, Rita Demetriou-Swanwick
Development Editor: Sally Davies
Project Manager: Mahalakshmi Nithyanand
Designer: Charles Gray
Illustrator: Graeme Chambers
Illustrations Manager: Merlyn Harvey

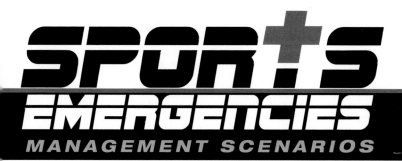

SPORTS EMERGENCIES

MANAGEMENT SCENARIOS

Edited by

John M O'Byrne, MCh FRCSI FRCS (Ortho) FFSEM(I) FFSEM(UK)
Abraham Colles Professor of Orthopaedic and Trauma Surgery, Department of Orthopaedic and Trauma Surgery, Royal College of Surgeons in Ireland at Cappagh National Orthopaedic Hospital, Dublin, Ireland

Brian M Devitt, MD MMedSc MRCSI
Department of Orthopaedic and Trauma Surgery, Royal College of Surgeons in Ireland at Cappagh National Orthopaedic Hospital, Dublin, Ireland

Foreword by Mr Raymond Moran

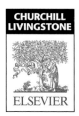

CHURCHILL
LIVINGSTONE

ELSEVIER

Edinburgh London New York Oxford Philadelphia St Louis Sydney Toronto 2010

CHURCHILL
LIVINGSTONE
ELSEVIER

ISBN: 978 0443 06865 2

1 British Library Cataloguing in Publication Data
A catalogue record for this book is available from the British Library

2 Library of Congress Cataloging in Publication Data
A catalog record for this book is available from the Library of Congress

Notices
Knowledge and best practice in this field are constantly changing. As new research and experience broaden our understanding, changes in research methods, professional practices, or medical treatment may become necessary.

Practitioners and researchers must always rely on their own experience and knowledge in evaluating and using any information, methods, compounds, or experiments described herein. In using such information or methods they should be mindful of their own safety and the safety of others, including parties for whom they have a professional responsibility.

With respect to any drug or pharmaceutical products identified, readers are advised to check the most current information provided (i) on procedures featured or (ii) by the manufacturer of each product to be administered, to verify the recommended dose or formula, the method and duration of administration, and contraindications. It is the responsibility of practitioners, relying on their own experience and knowledge of their patients, to make diagnoses, to determine dosages and the best treatment for each individual patient, and to take all appropriate safety precautions.

To the fullest extent of the law, neither the Publisher nor the editors or contributors, assume any liability for any injury and/or damage to persons or property as a matter of products liability, negligence or otherwise, or from any use or operation of any methods, products, instructions, or ideas contained in the material herein.

Printed in China

Contents

Foreword

I am delighted to write the foreword for this very practical and well presented manual on how to look after sports emergencies when they occur. There is great expertise and there have been great advances in the treatment of sports injuries in terms of surgical technique, non-surgical technique and in rehabilitation.

However, the care to the injured athlete from the moment of injury to their arrival at a specialist unit is crucial.

This book gives very practical advice in a very clearly presented way on how to look after an injured athlete during this initial phase. Not recognising the severity of an injury, or mismanaging an injury can make the injury worse and this can occasionally have catastrophic consequences.

The attraction of this book is not just the information but also the way it is presented. It is written by specialists, but presented in a way that should be understood by sports people, coaches, referees and also healthcare specialists. It outlines different scenarios that may arise and what should be done and also what should not be done.

It also gives a useful guide to that difficult question as to whether it is reasonable for a player to continue playing and also highlights that fact familiar to many involved in sports, that the players themselves are not always in the best position to make that decision.

Clearly, at elite levels of sport, there are teams of professionals that can respond to injuries. However, this represents a small percentage of people who participate in sports and unfortunately, recreational sports people do also suffer sports injuries and very occasionally sports emergencies.

This book is not a substitute for a proper accredited First-Aid course, but is a useful and reassuring guide to include in the kit bag for quick reference should you encounter a sports injury or emergency.

Mr Ray Moran MCh FRCSI
Medical Director
Sports Surgery Clinic
Dublin Ireland

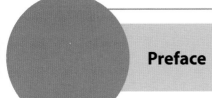

Preface

Sport is for everyone! Sport at any level is an extremely enjoyable and rewarding experience, whether you are a Sunday league soccer player or an international athlete. Participation in sport contributes to your physical, mental and emotional well-being.

However, injuries do occur. These are usually minor and incidental but on occasion they can be serious and cause permanent disability or even death.

Encountering injuries on the field of play is a stressful and nerve-racking experience for the injured player and also for those around who wish to help. This book is designed to provide clear directions to those who encounter an injured player.

These instructions will help people look after the player from the point of injury to the sideline and in particular will help the reader:

- to recognize the severity of the injury (Red, Amber, Green)
- to know what *can* and *should* be done
- to know what should *not* be done

The book is *not* a substitute for first-aid courses or dedicated training but should be used as a reminder of the important steps that should already have been learned. It is not intended to be a definitive emergency guide but instead an easy-to-use on-field manual.

February 2009

John M O'Byrne
Brian M Devitt

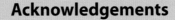

Acknowledgements

The editors would like to particularly thank Ursula Gormally for her tireless input and dedication in the preparation of this book.

Also thanks to Geraldine Taaffe of the Shamrock gift company for her creative contribution.

The figures and photographs below have been reproduced with permission of the copyright holders and are credited as follows:

Figure 11.6: McCrory P, Johnston K, Meeuwisse W et al, *Summary and agreement statement of the 2nd International Conference on Concussion in Sport*, Prague 2004, Concussion in Sport Group.

Figure 20.3: courtesy of patfalvey.com

Page 5, Sportsfile
Page 6, David Maher, Sportsfile
Page 8, Pat Murphy, Sportsfile
Page 13, Damien Eagers, Sportsfile
Page 17, Brian Lawless, Sportsfile
Page 19, Sportsfile
Page 39, Brian Lawless, Sportsfile
Page 42, David Maher, Sportsfile
Page 56, David Maher, Sportsfile
Page 61, Brendan Moran, Sportsfile
Page 66, David Maher, Sportsfile
Page 70, Damien Eagers, Sportsfile
Page 75, photographs of Ruby Walsh reproduced with the permission of Tom Burke and the Irish Independent
Page 89, Pat Murphy, Sportsfile
Page 91, Brendan Moran, Sportsfile
Page 114, David Maher, Sportsfile
Page 118, Paul Mohan, Sportsfile
Page 122, Damien Eagers, Sportsfile
Page 123, Brendan Moran, Sportsfile

Page 146, Damien Eagers, Sportsfile
Page 169, Brendan Moran, Sportsfile
Page 180, Ray McManus, Sportsfile
Page 185, Brendan Moran, Sportsfile
Page 211, Sportsfile

Dedications

To my parents, Ruth and Joe O'Byrne, my brother, Jim, and my sisters, Elizabeth, Ruth, Patricia and Mary.

John M O'Byrne

To my grandfathers, Brian McEvoy and Paddy Devitt, my family, and my wife, Marina.

Brian M Devitt

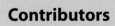

Contributors

Ciaran Bolger FRCSI(SN) PhD
Professor, Clinical Neuroscience and Chairman, National Department of Neurosurgery, Beaumont Hospital, Dublin, Ireland

Joseph S Butler MRCSI
Specialist Registrar in Trauma & Orthopaedic Surgery, Department of Trauma & Orthopaedic Surgery, Royal College of Surgeons in Ireland, Cappagh National Orthopaedic Hospital, Dublin, Ireland

Alan Byrne MRCPI MSc(sports and exercise) FFSEM
Medical Director of the Football Association of Ireland; Team Doctor to the Republic of Ireland Soccer Team; Sports Medicine Consultant and General Practitioner (Dublin)

Ann-Maria Byrne MA MB BCh LRCSPI MRCSI
Specialist Registrar, Trauma and Orthopaedics, Department of Orthopaedics, Cappagh National Orthopaedic Hospital, Dublin, Ireland

Kevin D Carson BSc(Hons) MB BS FFARCSI FFPMCAI FJFICMI
Consultant in Anaesthesia and Intensive Care Medicine; Clinical Director of Intensive Care and Director, Department of Anaesthesia, Intensive Care and Pain Medicine, Children's University Hospital, Dublin, Ireland

Frank Coffey MB DCH MMedSci DipSportsMed MRCPI FRCSEd FCEM
Consultant in Emergency Medicine, Nottingham University Hospitals NHS Trust; Nottingham Forest; Associate Professor, University of Nottingham, Nottingham, UK

Brian M Devitt MD MMedSc MRCSI
Specialist Registrar in Trauma and Orthopaedics, Cappagh National Orthopaedic Hospital, Dublin, Ireland

Frank Devitt BE PhD
Head, Department of Design and Innovation, School of Business and Law, National University of Ireland Maynooth, Maynooth, Ireland

Patrick Devitt MRCPsych
Consultant Psychiatrist, Mental Health Commission, St Martins House, Dublin, Ireland

Nicholas Eustace MB MMedSci FCA RCSI
Consultant Anaesthetist, Department of Anaesthesia, Cappagh National Orthopaedic Hospital, Dublin, Ireland

Stephen J Eustace MB MSc Rad Sci MRCPI FFR(RCSI) FRCR FFSEM
Newman Professor, Consultant Musculoskeletal Radiologist, Cappagh National Orthopaedic and Mater Misericordiae Hospitals, Dublin, Ireland

Eanna Falvey MB MRSPI MMedSc(Sports & Exercise) MFSEM
Sports Medicine Fellow, Department of Rheumatology, Sport and Exercise Medicine, Cork University Hospital, Cork, Ireland

Sean P Gaine MD PhD FRCPI FCCP FFSEM
Consultant Respiratory Physician, Mater Misericordiae University Hospital; Chief Medical Officer, Olympic Council of Ireland, Dublin, Ireland

Robert F Harrold BSc HDE MScEd
Director of Adult Education and Senior Biology Teacher, Malahide Community School, Dublin, Ireland

Gareth Horgan MB BCh MRCPI
Gastroenterology Specialist Registrar, Mater Misericordiae University Hospital, Dublin, Ireland

Fiona Kearns MB BCh BAO DCH DO
Medical Ophthalmic Physician, Beaumont Hospital, Dublin, Ireland

Ian P Kelly MCh FRCSI FRCS(Tr & Orth)
Consultant Orthopaedic Surgeon, Department of Orthopaedic Surgery, Waterford Regional Hospital, Waterford, Ireland

Paddy J Kenny MB BCh BAO FRCSI FRCS(Tr & Orth) MFSEM
Consultant Orthopaedic Surgeon, Cappagh National Orthopaedic Hospital, Dublin, Ireland

Garrett O Lawlor MB MRCPI
Specialist Registrar in Gastroenterology, Mater Misericordiae University Hospital, Dublin, Ireland

Conor McCarthy MD FRCPI FFSEM
Medical Director, Irish Rugby Football Union; Senior Clinical Lecturer, University College of Dublin; Consultant Rheumatologist, Mater Misericordiae University Hospital, Dublin, Ireland

Damian McCormack BSc(Hons) FRCSI FRCS(Orth) MCh
Clinical Professor of Orthopaedic Surgery, Mater Private Hospital, Dublin, Ireland

Gerry McEntee MCh FRCSI
Consultant Hepatobiliary and Pancreatic Surgeon, Mater Misericordiae University, Dublin, Ireland

Liam Moggan
Coach Education Development Officer, Coaching Ireland, University of Limerick, Limerick, Ireland

John H Mullett FRCS(Tr & Orth) MCh
Consultant Orthopaedic Surgeon, Beaumont Hospital and Cappagh National Orthopaedic Hospital, Dublin; Sports Surgery Clinic, Santry, Ireland

Ciaran Murray BSc Physio Hons MISCP
Chartered Physiotherapist, Private Practice, County Louth, Ireland

Jim O'Byrne
Team Leader, London, United Kingdom

John M O'Byrne MCh FRCSI FRCS (Ortho) FFSEM(I) FFSEM(UK)
Abraham Colles Professor of Orthopaedic and Trauma Surgery, Department of Orthopaedic and Trauma Surgery, Royal College of Surgeons in Ireland at Cappagh National Orthopaedic Hospital, Dublin, Ireland

Pat O'Neill MD MSc(Orth) DipSportsMed(London) FFSEM(I) FFSEM(UK)
Consultant in Orthopaedic and Sports Medicine, Mater Private Hospital; Dublin; Lecturer in Sports Medicine, Trinity College, Dublin, Ireland

Gary C O'Toole BSc(Hons) MB BAO BCh(Hons) MCh FRCS (Tr & Orth)
Consultant Orthopaedic Surgeon, St Vincent's University Hospital and Cappagh National Orthopaedic Hospital, Dublin, Ireland

Ashley R Poynton MD FRCSI FRCS(Tr & Orth)
Consultant Spinal Surgeon, National Spinal Injuries Unit, Mater Hospital, Dublin, Ireland

Joseph M Queally MRCSI
Registrar in Trauma and Orthopaedic Surgery, Royal College of Surgeons in Ireland, Cappagh National Orthopaedic Hospital, Dublin, Ireland

Ian Robertson MB BCh BAO MRCSI
Orthopaedic Registrar, Cappagh National Orthopaedic Hospital, Dublin, Ireland

Martin J Shelly MB BCh BAO BMedSc MRCSI
Specialist Registrar in Radiology, Department of Radiology, Mater Misericordiae University Hospital, Dublin, Ireland

Keith Synnott MB BCh BAO FRCSI(Tr & Orth)
Consultant Orthopaedic Surgeon, Department of Orthpaedic Surgery, Mater Misericordiae University Hospital, Dublin, Ireland

Mihai H Vioreanu MRCSI MCh(Orth)
Specialist Registrar in Trauma and Orthopaedic Surgery, Cappagh National Orthopaedic Hospital, Dublin, Ireland

James Walsh MCh MRCSI MB BAO LRCPI Dip(Man)
Specialist Registrar in Trauma and Orthopaedic Surgery, Cappagh National Orthopaedic Hospital, Dublin, Ireland

How to use this book

This book is primarily designed to provide clear instructions on how to deal with an injured player on the field of play. It is written in a simple stepwise manner with very little medical jargon and plenty of illustrations. We have divided the book into four sections.

Section 1 *Before* **the Game**. We discuss the factors that should be in place before the game to limit the occurrence of injuries. This section describes measures to prevent injury and preparations to deal with emergencies.

Section 2 *During* **the Game.** In the first few chapters of Section 2, we deal with the very important topics of life-threatening emergencies and immediate steps that should be taken. These are followed by chapters giving general guidelines about problems involving skin, muscle, tendon and bone.

Section 3 Where is the injury? Each of the chapters in Section 3 deals with a separate part of the body. When you have identified what part of the athlete's body is affected, go to the relevant chapter. Emergencies that occur with water sports or mountaineering are outlined at the end of the section.

Section 4 *After* **the Game**. We highlight the importance of assessing how the injury occurred. Could it have been avoided by better preparation? Was the injury dealt with properly? What do we do to improve care in the future?

When encountering an injury, the first priority is to decide whether it is serious and needs urgent hospitalization, whether it is moderate and the player needs to be substituted or whether it is minor and the player can continue. In order to achieve this we have colour-coded the injuries based on how serious they are.

- **Red Zone – a serious injury that requires urgent hospitalization.**

- Amber Zone – a moderate+ injury that requires further assessment, usually on the sideline. This may be subsequently re-zoned into Red or **Green**.

- **Green Zone – a minor knock or injury that can usually be treated on the field of play and the player can continue to participate.**

The first step in dealing with an injury on the field of play is to assess the player and decide into which zone the injury fits. We therefore start each subject with a section entitled 'What should I check for?' which outlines a list of steps which should be performed following the simple acronym SPORTS.

- **S**peak to the player – ask the player relevant questions regarding the injury to assess the severity
- **P**roblem identification – based on the answers to the questions and how the injury happened, it may be possible to identify the problem
- **O**bserve – the first step in physical examination is to look at the injured area and compare it to the normal side. Observe for anything usual, such as a deformity, skin abrasions, bleeding, lumps and bumps, etc
- **R**ule out serious injury – before proceeding any further, it is vital that you establish that the player does not have a serious injury which may threaten life or limb
- **T**ouch for tenderness – having put on gloves, you may now gently touch the injured area to assess for swelling, tenderness, the possibility of a pulled muscle, strained ligament or even broken bone
- **S**kills assessment – once the player has been assessed, a big factor in deciding whether they can play on is if they are able to perform the skills needed to participate in the game, e.g. if a tennis player falls on her shoulder, is she then able to swing her racket above her head? If not, she should come off!

Having recognized the injury, there are a number of things that you should and should not do. The next section in each chapter highlights 'What should I do?'. Once again, there are a number of simple instructions, which follow the acronym TREAT.

- **T**alk to the player – it is very important to speak with the player and explain what is going on and what you are doing. An injury may be very frightening and the player needs reassurance that they are being cared for. In some situations, it is not always clear whether the injury is in the amber zone or the green zone. In this case, it is reasonable to ask the player 'Do you think you can play on?'. Players normally know their own limitations

- **R**emove the player safely from the field of play – all red and amber zone injuries should be removed from the field of play in a controlled and safe manner, using appropriate equipment and personnel. In order to properly assess a player who may need to be substituted, it is easier and safer to perform the assessment on the sideline rather than on the field of play. Green zone injuries can be dealt with on the pitch or on the sideline, depending on the scenario

- **E**mergency transfer – all red zone injuries should be transferred to hospital as soon as possible. Life- and limb-threatening injuries should go by ambulance immediately with medical supervision. Other injuries should be taken to hospital by the quickest means available

- **A**void further injury – this section gives instructions on 'What should I *not* do?' to prevent further injury

- **T**reatment – this section provides definitive treatment for specific injuries and illustrated instructions on how to apply a neck collar, splint a broken leg, etc

At the beginning of each chapter there is a list of which injuries fall into the various zones. Following the basic instructions of 'What should I check for?' and 'What should I do?', specific injuries are dealt with separately with individual instructions.

It is impossible to cover all injury scenarios that may occur. However, we feel that by following these instructions, most injuries can be dealt with efficiently and effectively, allowing the game to continue and getting the athlete back playing safely as soon as possible.

Before the Game

Preparing to play

Fail to prepare, prepare to fail!

There are a number of factors that should be considered before taking part in sport to reduce the risk of injury to the player. The player must be physically, mentally and technically prepared before participating. Equally important is the role of the coach, the medical team and the officials to ensure the game is played safely and injuries are dealt with properly and quickly. In this chapter we consider how everybody involved should prepare.

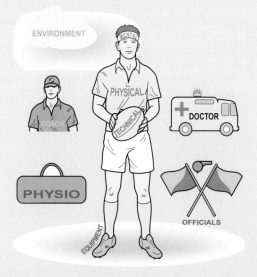

chapter 1

The coach

L Moggan, R Harrold

Coaches play a crucial role in sport. They are responsible for training players in a sport by analyzing their performances, instructing in relevant skills and by providing encouragement. Yet, the role of the coach is not just coaching. The responsibility for player welfare lies with the coach, and frequently the coach is called upon to manage injuries in the absence of trained medical personnel. As such, it is recommended that the coach should complete a first aid course prior to taking up a coaching position.

In this chapter, some important issues related to the coach's role in player welfare are discussed.

PLAYERS

Are the players carrying an injury?

- The closer it gets to a game, the less prepared many players are to make a call on an injury. So you, the coach, will have to

Do they have a proper diet?

- Have they eaten too much or too little prior to their event?
- What steps have they taken to prevent dehydration?

Are they fit?

- Proper warm-up can prevent injury
- Are they under the influence of drugs?
- Are they mentally OK?
- Have they had appropriate technical preparation, e.g. rugby tackling, diving?
- Is the opposition appropriately matched, especially in contact sports such as rugby? How do you know?
- Ensure warm-down after the event

OTHER FACTORS

- Examine the equipment, environment and facilities
- Rules must be understood and applied
- Ensure the athlete wants to play and enjoys participating
- Vary training and make it safe, fun and relevant

THE COACH'S BAG

While a well-stocked first aid bag is essential, we must take care to avoid complicating potentially stressful situations. A simple rule of thumb may clarify matters for those kitting out a first aid bag: 'If you don't understand what it is and what it does, don't have it in your bag!' The following list is a good start and can be added to as your experience increases. Always remember to check your bag regularly as it will quickly become depleted, often unbeknownst to you!

- Ice pack
- Water bottle
- Gauze swabs
- Nasal packing
- Tape, tape cutter
- Petroleum jelly
- Sudocrem
- Gauze pads, various sizes
- Adhesive skin closures
- Tincture of benzoin
- Irrigation solution (normal saline, eyewash)
- Elastic adhesive bandage (2.5 cm, 5 cm)
- Compression bandage (5 cm, 7.5 cm, 10 cm)
- Triangular bandage
- Adhesive dressings (e.g. Primapore, OpSite)
- Antiseptic ointment/spray (e.g. Betadine, Savlon)
- Melolin dressings ×12
- Skin-care pad (e.g. 2nd Skin, Compeed)
- List of players' contacts and telephone numbers
- Laminated card with telephone number of local hospital and emergency services

chapter 2

The medical team

C Murray, P O'Neill

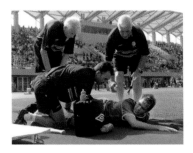

A critical aspect of success in sports relates to the time spent training and practising. This theory is equally applicable in providing medical assistance and is particularly relevant when dealing with emergency scenarios: airway, breathing, circulation, neck stabilization, and player transfer. A medical team that has rehearsed the various scenarios that may arise on the field of play prior to the event will be much more effective and efficient in dealing with a situation if it occurs.

This book is *not* a substitute for a course in emergency management but is a reminder of steps you should take in the stressful situation of dealing with an injury on the field of play. It is mandatory to have undertaken specific training in these techniques.

KNOW YOUR TEAM!

A list of all emergency phone numbers should be readily available:

- Local doctor
- Local accident and emergency room
- Ambulance
- Local dentist
- Fire Brigade

Familiarize yourself with techniques and practise as a team. Each member of the team should know their roles in an emergency scenario.

Know your players – medical conditions, injuries, etc. Player welfare is more important than winning.

Appropriate equipment should be available and in good

condition. The following lists give suggestions for the contents of the physiotherapist's bag and the team medical bag.

THE PHYSIOTHERAPIST'S BAG

- Ice pack and wet towel
- Cold compress/cold wipe
- Crepe bandages: 7.5 cm and 10 cm
- Water bottle/fluids
- Protective gloves
- Orthopaedic shears/scissors
- Airway and face mask
- Quick-drying adherent spray/ skin toughener
- Pretaping underwrap
- Adhesive Elastoplast support bandages 7.5 cm and 10 cm
- Zinc oxide tape 2.5 cm and 5 cm
- Adhesive orthopaedic felt
- Ribbon gauze (2.5 cm) tie-ups
- Gauze swabs – sterile
- Petroleum jelly
- Topical irrigation solution
- Antiseptic ointment/spray
- Cotton wool balls – sterile
- Adhesive surgical dressing (Mepore)
- Adhesive skin closures
- Paraffin gauze dressing – sterile

- Fabric Elastoplast strip
- Mefix/Hypafix adhesive dressing 10 cm
- Nasal sponges
- Eyewash
- Blister kit: 2nd Skin-type gel, Compeed, gel-lined digital caps
- Chiropody nail pliers and emery board
- Light insole (cut to size)
- Triangular bandage and pins
- Mallet finger splint
- Soap
- Paracetamol (acetaminophen)
- Nasal decongestant
- Smelling salts
- Massage oil/creams
- Freeze spray

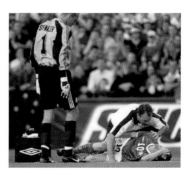

MEDICAL BAG

This bag should be available to the team for all matches and should be familiar to coaches, physios, and the backroom team – even if there is no physician in attendance.

- Ice pack
- Cryo/Cuff
- Water bottle
- Examination gloves
- Ice freeze
- Gauze swabs
- Nasal packing/nasal tampons
- Tape cutter
- Adhesive skin closures

Taping

- Skin toughner
- Toughner remover
- Pre-taping protective tape (e.g. Fixomull/Hypafix)
- Rigid sports tape (2.5 cm, 3.8 cm, 5 cm) (e.g. Leukotape/ Mueller M Tape)
- Elastic adhesive bandage (2.5 cm, 5 cm)
- Adhesive felt
- Orthopaedic support foam (e.g. Leukofoam)
- Compression bandage (5 cm, 7.5 cm, 10 cm)
- Cylindrical elastic support (e.g. Tubigrip)

Wound care

- Gauze pads, various sizes
- Tape, tape cutter
- Adhesive skin closures
- Tincture of benzoin
- Irrigation solution (physiological saline, eyewash)
- Compression bandage
- Alcohol swabs
- Skin care pad (e.g. 2nd Skin, Compeed)
- Adhesive dressings (e.g. Primapore, OpSite)
- Antiseptic ointment/spray (e.g. Betadine, Savlon)
- Melolin dressings ×12
- Sudocrem

Orthopaedic/neurological

- Cervical collar (adjustable)
- Guedel airway and face mask
- Triangular bandage/shoulder sling
- Extremity splints (fibreglass with padding, malleable aluminium, air, vacuum)
- Crutches
- Joint support braces
- Heel lifts
- Arch supports
- Temporary orthotics/insoles

General

- Towel
- Arnica

- Massage oil
- Topical anti-inflammatory
- Nail clippers/pliers/emery board
- Nail brush
- Mirror
- Cotton buds
- Safety pins
- Pen and notebook
- Warm clothing
- Blankets
- Raingear
- Milton sterilising tablets/liquid
- Icebox

CHECKLIST OF EQUIPMENT AND SUPPLIES FOR THE TEAM PHYSICIAN

While 'Be prepared' must always be our motto, there is no such thing as 'the complete list' for a team physician's bag: each sport and team will have its specific requirements and desires. Consequently, your bag will be a

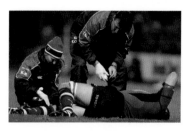

work in progress, something that will grow with you as your experience increases. What follows is a good start, but make sure you add to it constantly. Some emergency equipment – e.g. defibrillators, ACLS medications, orthopaedic equipment – will be available in an ambulance. It is important to liase with the ambulance service before a game to check what they have.

On person

- Examination gloves
- Gauze pads
- Petroleum jelly
- Adhesive tape
- Nasal packing/nasal tampons
- Trauma shears
- Pocket cardiopulmonary resuscitation mask
- Pen and paper
- Penlight
- Cotton buds
- Pocket knife/multi-tool
- Mobile phone/radio
- Smelling salts

Wound care kit

- Gauze pads, various sizes
- Tape, tape cutter
- Adhesive tape, various sizes, rigid/elastic

- Astringent (e.g. hydrogen peroxide)
- Topical antibiotic ointment
- Adhesive skin closures
- Tincture of benzoin
- Irrigation solution (normal saline, eyewash)
- Compression bandage
- Alcohol swabs
- Skin care pad (2nd Skin, Compeed)

Suture kit

- Lidocaine (1%, with and without adrenaline (epinephrine)
- Syringes and needles
- Sterile gloves, sterile fields
- Sterilizing solution (povidone-iodine)
- Disposable suture tray
- Suture (absorbable and non-absorbable)
- Sharps container
- Suture clips and remover
- Scalpel/scalpel blades

Eye kit

- Eye patches
- Petroleum-impregnated swabs (Jelonet) to aid eye closure
- Fluorescein drops with/without lidocaine

- Eyewash
- Blue light
- Topical antibiotic drops/ointment
- Tape
- Contact lens container

Nasal kit

- Nasal packing – ribbon gauze
- Nasal tampons
- Packing impregnated with:
  - adrenaline (epinephrine) (1:200)
  - framycetin sulphate (Soframycin) ointment

Sideline diagnosis

- Blood-pressure cuff
- Stethoscope
- Otoscope/ophthalmoscope
- Reflex hammer
- Glucometer (with lancets and test strips)
- Cognitive function screen (Maddock's Questionnaire)
- Tongue depressor
- Sports concussion assessment tool (SCAT)

Neurological/orthopaedic

(These are normally provided by the ambulance service – liaise prior to event.)

- Rigid backboard with body/ head straps
- Head immobilization devices
- Oral airway
- Face mask removal tools
- Knee immobilizer
- Crutches Finger splints (aluminium/foam)
- Extremity splints (fibreglass with padding, malleable aluminium, air, vacuum)
- Triangular bandage/shoulder sling

Medications

- Oral analgesics:
  - Paracetamol (acetaminophen) (500 mg tabs)
  - Ibuprofen (600 mg tabs)
  - Codeine phosphate
- Injectable analgesics:
  - Tramadol hydrochloride
  - Morphine
  - Pethidine
- Antacid
- Proton pump inhibitor (e.g. pantoprazole)
- Antispasmodic (e.g. hyoscine butylbromide)
- Oral decongestant (e.g. pseudoephedrine)
- Nasal decongestant spray (e.g. xylometazoline or beclometasone)
- Olbas Oil
- Antihistamine: sedating (e.g. chlorpheniramine), non-sedating (e.g. loratadine)
- Antitussive syrup (e.g. codeine phosphate)
- Mucolytic syrup (e.g. carbocysteine)
- Throat lozenges
- Antidiarrhoeal (e.g. loperamide)
- Antiemetic (e.g. metoclopramide, oral/ intramuscular)
- Glucose (tabs, paste or gel)
- Nitroglycerin sublingual spray
- Ear drops (cerumenolytic/ antibiotic/corticosteroid)
- Sedatives (e.g. zolpidem)
- Muscle relaxant (e.g. diazepam)
- Oral contraceptive pill
- Tetanus toxoid
- Faecal softener
- Creams/ointments:
  - Antifungal
  - Antibiotic
  - Corticosteroid
  - Anti-inflammatory
- Antibiotics:
  - Co-amoxiclav
  - Clarithromycin
  - Flucloxacillin

- Benzylpenicillin
- Ciprofloxacillin
- Bronchodilators (e.g. salbutamol, budesonide)
- Oral prednisolone
- Oral antiviral (e.g. famciclovir)
- Electrolyte replacement sachets (e.g. Dioralyte)

Anaphylaxis kit

- Adrenaline (Anapen)
- Hydrocortisone (+ water for solution)
- Prochlorperazine

Airway management

- Endotracheal tubes with stylet
- Oral airways
- Laryngoscope (with blades, light source)
- Syringes
- Lubricant
- Cricothyrotomy kit

Breathing

- Bag-valve-mask (various)
- Suction device

Circulatory support

- Intravenous catheters and tubing
- Intravenous solutions (physiological saline; 5% dextrose)

Drugs: ACLS medications

(Normally provided by cardiac ambulance – liaise prior to game.)

- Atropine (prefilled 1 mg syringes)
- Adrenaline (epinephrine) 1:1000 (prefilled 1 mg syringes)
- Lidocaine (prefilled 100 mg syringes)
- Lidocaine intravenous drip solution (E)
- Sodium bicarbonate (prefilled syringe)
- Dextrose 50% (prefilled 50 ml syringe)
- Nitroglycerin spray
- Aspirin 300 mg
- Oxygen tank, masks, tubing

Electrical monitoring

- Cardiac monitor/defibrillator

General/miscellaneous

- Ice packs
- Urine reagent strips
- Sunscreen
- Penknife/multi-tool – Swiss army knife
- Safety pins
- List of banned substances
- Dental rolls
- Dental kit (cyanoacrylate, transport media)

- Pen and paper
- Flashlight and batteries
- Mirror
- Prescription pad
- Consent forms
- Pre-printed information forms
- Warm clothing
- Blankets
- Rain wear
- Copy of medical licences

DRUGS IN SPORT/ BANNED SUBSTANCES

The combination of increasing governing body drug testing and the number of supplements/ ergogenic agents available to athletes has made this area a minefield. Always check if in doubt **before** prescribing. The Monthly Index of Medical Specialities (MIMS) has an extremely handy method of 'flagging' contraband products. Helplines for information in various countries are as follows:

- Ireland: +353 1 8608800/ www.irishsportscouncil.ie
- Australia: +61 6206 0200/ www.asada.gov.au
- Canada: +1 800 672 7775/ www.cces.ca
- New Zealand: 0 800 DRUGFREE (0800 378 437)/ nasda@nzsda.co.nz
- South Africa: +27 (0)21 6837129/ drugfree@iafrica.com
- United Kingdom: +44 (0)20 7211 5100/drug-free@uksport.gov.uk
- United States: +1 816 474-8655/ info@drugfreesport.com

The player

B M Devitt, P Devitt

A fit player is better than an injured star!

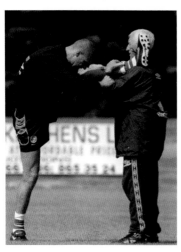

- A player suffering from illness should be reviewed by trained medical personnel before taking part
- The general rule applies – do not play if you have a temperature
- Any player participating with a pre-existing injury runs the risk of making the injury worse, causing more serious harm
- A player who plays with an injury is often less mentally prepared and often underperforms

PHYSICAL PREPARATION

- The player should have a basic level of fitness to take part in the game
- The player should be trained in the techniques of the individual sport
- A warm-up before the sport is advised to reduce the risk of injury

MENTAL PREPARATION

Get your mind on the game!

Mental preparation is crucial to improve performance and to reduce risk of injury. Sport is a highly charged, emotional experience where normally sensible people can lose control of themselves. In such a situation, players are more likely to cause harm to themselves or others.

Let us look now at the positive and negative factors involved in getting your mind on the game.

Positive factors

- Focus: on goals, technique, strategy, desire
- Motivation: the will to succeed, the desire to achieve your goals

An ideal mental approach to sport involves 'the five Cs':

- Calmness
- Confidence
- Courage
- Control
- Clarity

Teams can often be found reciting these as a mantra!

I've got butterflies in my tummy, what do I do?

Players often describe the feeling of nerves before a game. Anxiety may be a good thing and is known to improve performance. However, too much anxiety, particularly on a big occasion, can cause a player to become paralysed with fear. This process is known as 'stage fright'.

Many athletes perform relaxation techniques prior to a game to reduce their anxiety and improve their focus, such as yoga, visualization, meditation.

Negative factors

- 'Stage fright'
- **Obsessive compulsive disorder** – indecisiveness caused by anxiety
- **Superstitions** – a form of compulsion that relieves anxiety, which may or may not be a good thing. If the means to fulfil the superstition are not available, this may be a guarantee of failure
- **Phobias** – irrational fears, such as relating to a particular 'bogey' team
- **Failure of mental preparation** causing failure of performance can lead to depression and vice versa. Look out for these tell-tale signs and get the player checked out by the doctor: poor sleep, loss of interest, guilt, energy, lack of concentration, overuse of alcohol, psychosis (delusions, hallucinations), suicidal ideation
- **Burnout** – this is often due to overtraining: 'All work and no play makes Jack a dull boy (or Jill a dull girl)'. It may be due to lack of variety in training: 'A change is as good as a rest'
- **Lack of perspective** – this can lead to overstress, which may

mean playing below par or loss of form. (It's only a game!) An example would be over-reaction to being dropped or being unable to play because of injury

- **Drug and substance abuse** – smelling of alcohol before a game or use of recreational drugs increases incidence of injury. Players should not be allowed to play in these circumstances and should be disciplined

- **Personality issues** – the 'hot head' may need counselling to improve performance. Consider substituting a player if there are personality issues – the player may incur the wrath of the referee and get a yellow or red card as a result. The 'lazy player' may need a more direct approach to motivation – 'a kick up the backside'!

Psychosomatic symptoms

These are physical symptoms due to stress, e.g. headache, chest pain, fast heart rate, stomach upset, diarrhoea, abdominal pain, dizziness.

This diagnosis should only be made by trained personnel when physical examination is clear and when a pattern of such symptoms has been noted previously.

MENTAL ILLNESS AND SPORT

Although it is not widely recognized, at least one in 10 sports participants suffers mental illness, the same proportion as the general population. Mental illness may be even more prevalent than this because of the emotional stress associated with sport. The common mental disorders are anxiety/depression, bipolar disorder (manic depressive illness) and schizophrenia. Before going on tour it is a good idea to screen for personal and family history of the serious mental disorders, especially manic depressive illness.

PSYCHOLOGICAL EMERGENCIES – WHAT SHOULD I DO?

The team doctor should be aware of any player on medication for a mental disorder. **Be aware of antidoping rules!** (See the WADA website: www.wada-ama.org.)

Panic

This may involve a feeling of imminent death – 'I thought I was having a heart attack'. First, it is important to rule out any physical cause of illness.

If the player is hyperventilating (fast, shallow breathing), get them to breathe into a paper bag.

- **Reassurance** – approach in a confident manner and talk the player down. 'It's only a panic attack, you won't die, you've had these before, you'll be OK in a few minutes and I guarantee you'll play the game of your life today!'

- **Relaxation** – focus on contracting major muscle groups in turn up to a count of 10 seconds and relaxing gradually for 10 seconds until the muscles are totally relaxed, e.g. get the player to clench their fist increasingly for 10 seconds and relax bit by bit for a further 10 seconds. While relaxing, eyes should be closed and the player is asked to repeat some 'positive affirmations', e.g. 'I'm fully prepared', 'I feel great!', 'Everything will be fine'

A doctor may want to give medication if the anxiety is very severe.

If the situation can't be helped off the field of play, the player should be accompanied to hospital.

Mania

This may manifest itself as socially inappropriate or risk-taking behaviour, little sleep, irritability, grandiosity (e.g. 'I am Jesus Christ – God has given me a mission to win the cup this year!'), over-talkativeness and poor judgement. It may be associated with alternating tears and hysterical laughter. **Ensure that the player is safe and seek urgent medical attention!**

Psychosis

Psychosis involves thinking or behaviour that is out of contact with reality. A sufferer may experience delusions (false beliefs, e.g. 'Aliens have put a microchip into my brain to control me'), hallucinations (hearing voices that are not present) or disorganized speech or behaviour. **Ensure that the player is safe and seek urgent medical attention!**

Come on ref! – role of the referee or official

F Devitt, Jim O'Byrne

Put player welfare above competition

Referees, although occasionally unpopular, are extremely important in sport. By refereeing a fair and balanced contest, they ensure player safety during a game. It is vital that the medical team and referee communicate before and during a game.

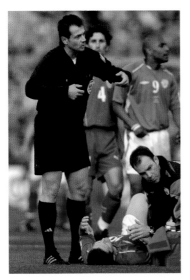

ROLE OF THE REFEREE OR OFFICIALS

- Apply the rules
- Prevent a mismatch
- Stop dangerous play
- Issue red/yellow card
- Monitor equipment/ facilities
- Stop play if a player is injured

ENVIRONMENT

- **The playing surface** – ensure that this is clear of obstacles (such as broken glass), even and well maintained
- **Weather conditions** – may have a big impact on the game. Extremes of heat and cold, rain, fog and ice can all increase the risk of injury. Where the risk to the players is too great, a decision should be made by the referee to postpone the competition

It takes a big person to make the right decision

EQUIPMENT

This can range from appropriate clothing (e.g. footwear) to equipment used by the athlete to perform the sport (vaulting pole, skis, bicycle, etc.). These should be appropriate and properly maintained.

During the game

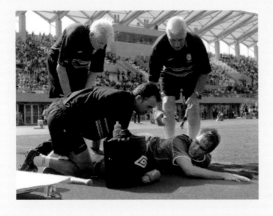

5

The ABC chapter

A M Byrne, N Eustace

A = Airway   B = Breathing   C = Circulation

This chapter is designed as a quick reference guide for those who have previously been instructed in basic life-saving techniques.

The aim of this chapter is to remind you how to:

- assess the collapsed athlete
- initiate basic life support to maintain blood and air flow
- use a defibrillator

 INFORMATION

Risks to the rescuer

- The rescuer's personal safety comes first
- Be aware of risks from the environment, e.g. attempting rescue and resuscitation in the water, on a mountainside, on a motor circuit
- Be aware of risks of infection from the person to be resuscitated. Wear gloves and use a pocket mask, if available.

REQUIREMENTS

Team

- Two rescuers
- Helpers for logrolling

Basic equipment

- Gloves
- Towel
- Scissors (to remove clothing)
- Razor (to shave chest)
- Face mask

Advanced equipment

- Guedel airway
- Ambu bag
- Nasopharyngeal airway
- Laryngeal mask airway
- Automated external defibrillator (AED)

A = AIRWAY

Step 1 (Fig. 5.1A)

- Is the athlete unconscious?
- Was there trauma? If yes, **stabilize neck** (see Ch. 7)
- Do not attempt to move the athlete
- Speak to the athlete – 'Are you OK? Where are you hurt?'

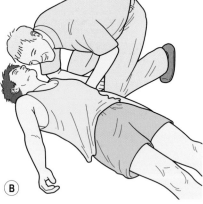

Fig. 5.1 Assessing the collapsed athlete. **A.** Step 1 – 'Hello, hello, hello! Open your eyes!'
B. Checking for breathing – look, feel, listen.

Step 2 (Fig. 5.1B)

- Check if the athlete is breathing normally
- If the patient can speak without hoarseness or wheeze, the airway is open
- If unconscious, remove anything that may be obstructing the airway, such as a mouthguard or broken teeth
- Using a gloved finger, sweep the tongue forwards from the back of the throat (**no finger sweep in children**)

Step 3 (Fig. 5.2)

- If unconscious, gently open the airway by tilting the chin upwards with one hand and pushing back on the forehead with the other hand (Fig. 5.2A)

OR

- If possibility of a neck injury, open the airway with a 'jaw thrust' by putting fingers behind the angle of the jaw and lifting the jaw upwards to open the mouth and airway (Fig. 5.2B)

If the athlete is face down, logrolling is required for airway access.

Clearing the airway takes priority over other injuries.

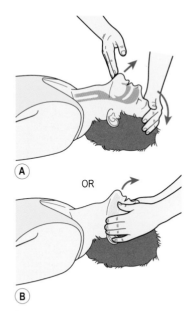

OR

Fig. 5.2 Opening the airway **A.** Chin lift. **B.** Jaw thrust.

If these methods successfully open the airway:

- Check for any other life-threatening injuries
- If no neck pain or possibility of spine injury, place in recovery position (Fig. 5.3)
- Wait with athlete for help to arrive
- If vomiting, see instructions on p. 27

If airway is open but spontaneous breathing does not occur, start by giving two breaths (see next section).

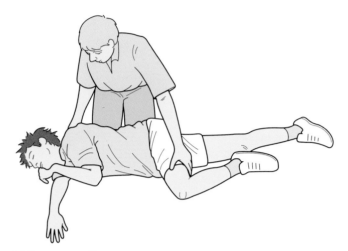

Fig. 5.3 The recovery position.

Placing the player in the recovery position

1. Place arm as shown in Figure 5.4A.
2. Bend opposite knee and bring across opposite hand (Fig. 5.4B).
3. Turn the player on their side (Fig. 5.4C).

Advanced techniques to protect airway

- To maintain the airway, an oropharyngeal or Guedel airway can be used. Select the appropriate size by placing the flange parallel to the front teeth – the tip of the airway should not go beyond the angle of the jaw (Fig. 5.5). If too long, it could actually obstruct the airway. If too short, it could push the tongue against the back of the throat and again obstruct the airway

- With gloved hands remove any foreign objects, e.g. mouthguard, from the mouth

- Open the mouth, gently pushing apart the upper and lower teeth

- Begin inserting the airway upside down, with the curved part toward the tongue to prevent pushing the tongue back into the throat (Fig. 5.6A)

- When the airway reaches the back of the tongue, rotate the device 180° so that the tip

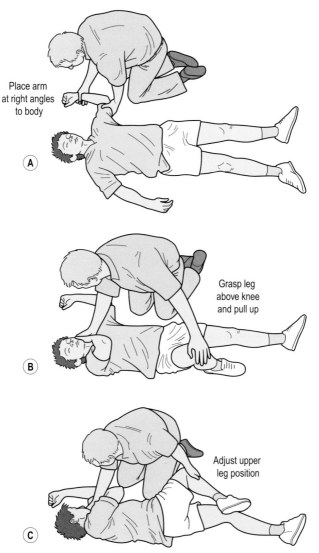

Place arm at right angles to body

A

Grasp leg above knee and pull up

B

Adjust upper leg position

C

Fig. 5.4 Placing the player in the recovery position. **A.** Place arm as shown. **B.** Bend opposite knee and bring opposite hand across. **C.** Turn the player on to their side.

points down as it approaches the back of the throat (Fig. 5.6B)

- If the athlete gags or appears to be gasping for air after insertion, remove the airway immediately

- Recheck the size before reinsertion

- If no spontaneous breathing or abnormal breathing occurs, start artificial ventilation using a mouth-to-mask or Ambu bag and mask (Figs 5.7–5.9)

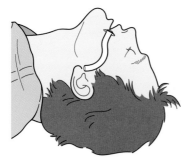

Fig. 5.5 Selecting the appropriate size of Guedel airway – measure from the corner of the mouth to the angle of the jaw. This distance correspomds to the appropriate size of airway.

> ### ⓘ INFORMATION
>
> **Advanced airway techniques**
>
> - Nasopharyngeal airway – avoid if athlete has a head injury
> - Laryngeal mask airway
> - Endotracheal tube
> - Emergency cricothyroidotomy
>
> All these interventions require advanced training. They should only be carried out by a qualified practitioner. The athlete needs immediate transfer to hospital for definitive treatment.

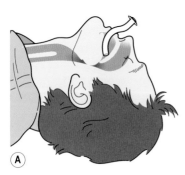
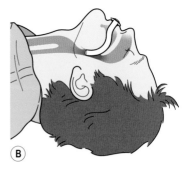

Ⓐ   Ⓑ

Fig. 5.6 Advanced airway. **A.** Introducing the Guedel airway. **B.** Rotate the Guedel airway through 180°.

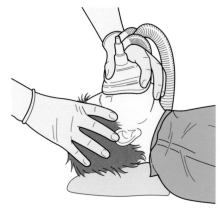

Fig. 5.7 Ambu bag ventilation using a mask. Ensure there is a seal with the mask around the player's mouth and nose.

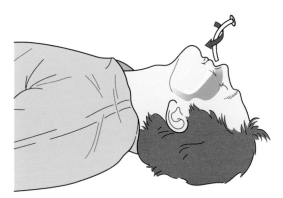

Fig. 5.8 Inserting a nasopharyngeal airway.

Vomiting

If there are no concerns about the spine and the athlete is vomiting, place in the recovery position. If there is concern about the spine, use the logrolling technique – see p. 27

B = BREATHING

Maintenance of open airway (A) is essential before proceeding to breathing (B) (Fig. 5.10).

• Look, listen and feel for signs of breathing

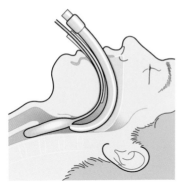

Fig. 5.9 Laryngeal mask airway.

- Look for signs of laboured breathing: flaring of nostrils, blueness around lips
- If no spontaneous breathing, give two rescue breaths
  - Mouth-to-mouth ventilation – rescuer seals athlete's mouth with their own mouth (Fig. 5.11), pinches the nose closed and then blows air into the mouth. Use a face mask where available

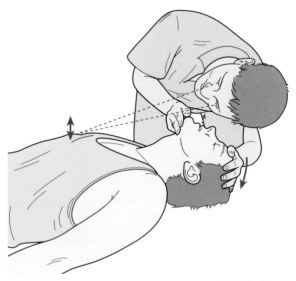

Fig. 5.10 Opening the airway. Tilt the head backward with one hand; lift the chin forward with your finger. Look, feel, listen for breathing. Prepare for breath.

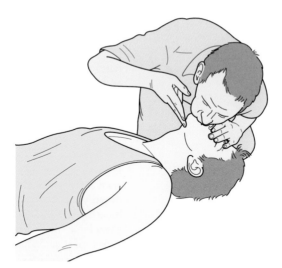

Fig. 5.11 Mouth to mouth breathing. If a mask is not available, take a deep breath in. Make a seal around the player's mouth with your own mouth and breathe out slowly.

- Mouth-to-nose ventilation – used if athlete has sustained facial injuries that prevent using the mouth. The rescuer closes the athlete's mouth, covers the nose with their mouth, breathes gently, then releases the jaw to allow exhalation
- Mouth-to-nose-and-mouth ventilation – used when resuscitating a child so that rescuer's mouth can cover and seal the child's nose and mouth

Use a pocket mask or protective facial sheet if available.

C = CIRCULATION

- Check for carotid pulse in the neck (Fig. 5.12)
- If you can feel it, continue rescue breaths until athlete starts breathing
- If no neck injury, turn the athlete into the recovery position
- After two rescue breaths, if the athlete is not breathing, check carotid pulse again

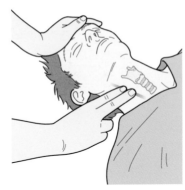

Fig. 5.12 Feeling for the carotid pulse. Feel over the airway with two fingers. Move your fingers outward, away from the midline. Press your fingers into the neck and feel for a pulsation.

Commence cardiopulmonary resuscitation (CPR)

Position hands for chest compressions

1. With the index and middle fingers of your lower hand, locate one of the casualty's lowermost ribs on the side nearer you. Slide your fingertips along the rib to the point at which it meets the breastbone. Place your middle finger at this point and the index finger beside it on the breastbone (Fig. 5.13)

2. Place the heel of your other hand on the breastbone and slide it down to meet your index finger. This is the point at which you will apply pressure (Fig. 5.14A)

3. Place the heel of your first hand on top of the other hand and interlock your fingers (Fig. 5.14B).

Give chest compressions and rescue breaths

1. Lean well over the player, with your arms straight. Press down vertically on the breastbone and depress the chest by about 4–5 cm (1.5–2 in) (Fig. 5.15)

2. Compress the chest 30 times, at a rate of 100 compressions per minute

3. Tilt the head, lift the chin and give two rescue breaths

4. Alternate 30 chest compressions with two rescue breaths.

 INFORMATION

If a person is not trained in CPR and is unable to give adequate breaths, then the person should provide hands-only CPR. The rescuer should continue with hands-only CPR until an automated external defibrillator arrives and is ready for use or trained personnel arrive and take over the victim. Likewise, if a person was previously trained in giving CPR, but is not confident in giving proper rescue breaths, hands-only CPR should be carried out. Hands-only CPR is continuous chest compressions at a rate of 100 compressions per minute.

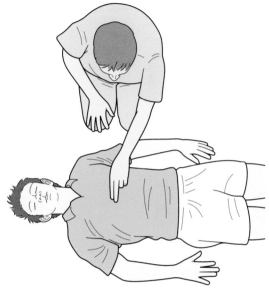

Fig. 5.13 Commencing CPR. Feel down the middle of the chest until you reach the end of the sternum – the position where the rib cages join. Pick a point two finger breaths above this point.

Continue resuscitation until help arrives

- Continue CPR until emergency help takes over, the casualty makes a movement or takes a breath, or you are too exhausted to continue
- After 30 chest compressions, give another two rescue breaths
- Continue at a ratio of 30 compressions to two breaths
- Recheck carotid pulse if the athlete moves or breathes spontaneously

If the athlete starts breathing again, place in recovery position and **wait until help arrives.**

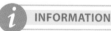 **INFORMATION**

If two rescuers are present

- Seeking help is the main priority
- Open and maintain airway as described above
- First rescuer gives two breaths followed by 30 compressions by second rescuer
- Continue resuscitation using this ratio of breaths to chest compressions.

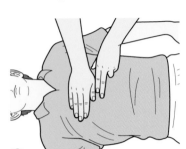

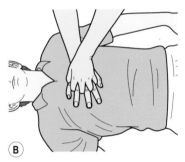

Fig. 5.14 Commence CPR. **A.** Slide heel of hand down. **B.** Interlock your fingers.

USE OF AN AUTOMATED EXTERNAL DEFIBRILLATOR

Athletes may collapse due to sudden cardiac arrest. Signs include:

• unresponsiveness

• no breathing activity

• no pulse

An AED can give an electric shock to restart the heart's natural rhythm. AEDs give verbal instructions to the rescuer and are available in many sports clubs, airports, shopping centres and factories. Look for the indication sign in Figure 5.16.

1. Check ABCs

2. Call for help and ask for the AED

3. Commence resuscitation using the ABC method

4. Check for a pulse

5. If there is no pulse, prepare the AED

6. Prepare the athlete by cutting off the shirt, drying the chest. Quickly shaving the chest hair may be required before attaching the AED electrode pads, to give a better contact

7. A second rescuer should continue resuscitation until the AED electrode pads are attached in the positions shown in Figure 5.17. The AED analyses the heart rhythm and will not fire unless it is appropriate

8. **Make sure no one is touching the athlete**

9. **Press the 'shock' button only if directed verbally by the AED**

10. Continue with resuscitation.

 INFORMATION

Always seek definitive medical help.

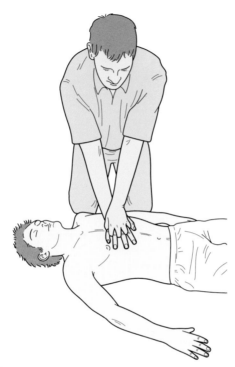

Fig. 5.15 Press down vertically with your elbows locked. Press down 4–5 cm.

Fig. 5.16 The symbol denoting a defibrillator.

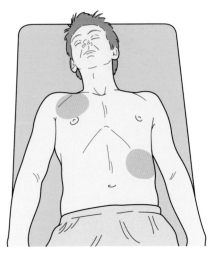

Fig. 5.17 Positioning of the defibrillator pads.

The collapsed player

B M Devitt, K D Carson

COLLAPSE WITH NO TRAUMA

This is a very serious event. Call for help immediately!

Red Zone
More likely to occur during a game.

- **Cardiac arrest**
- **Stroke**
- **Diabetes – insulin reaction or diabetic coma**
- **Severe asthma attack**

Amber Zone
More likely to occur after a game.

- Faint
- Exhaustion
- Dehydration

Green zone

- **Muscle or joint problems**

A collapsed player should be treated as a **Red Zone** or **Amber Zone** injury until proven otherwise. Remove them from the field of play and ensure they are assessed by trained medical personnel.

An athlete with collapse related to a muscle of joint problem can return to play only if they perform the necessary skills – see Chapter 9.

What do I check for?

If the player is unconscious and does not come around quickly, go immediately to the ABC chapter (p. 21)!

With any head injury, be aware of possible neck injury and protect the neck.

Speak to the player

- 'Hello, hello, can you hear me?'
- 'Open your eyes'
- 'What is your name?'
- 'Do you know where you are?'
- 'Are you in pain?'
- 'Can you tell me what happened?'
- 'Do you have any medical conditions?'
- 'Are you taking any drugs?'

If the player is drowsy – Ask anybody who saw the incident what happened?

Ask if there is anyone who knows the player?
Find out if they are on medication or have a medical condition

Problem identification
Always assume the worst-case scenario.
Did the collapse happen during or after the game?

Common causes of collapse during the game

Heart causes

Lethal arrhythmia (conduction problem)

Heart attack

Major vessel rupture (aortic dissection, aortic aneurysm)

Metabolic emergencies

Symptomatic Hyponatraemia (low salt)

Diabetic emergencies – Insulin Reaction (low blood sugar) or Diabetic Coma

Brain conditions

Stroke

Brain haemorrhage (Subarachnoid bleeding)

Seizure

Extremes of body temperature

Hyperthermia (overheating)

Hypothermia (Low body temperature)

Gasping for air

Extreme asthma attack

Anaphylactic reaction allergy

Aspirated a foreign body: Chunk of a sports bar, chewing gum or mouth guard

Severe cramping and other orthopaedic conditions

Common causes of collapse after the game

Exercise-associated collapse

Faint – Temporary Drop In Blood Pressure

Over heating

Dehydration

Severe cramping or other orthopaedic conditions

Is the player making sense?

Yes. Encouraging sign, less likely to be a serious head injury. Quiz the player about what happened.

• Do you know why you collapsed?

• Has this happened before?

• Do you have any medical problems?

• Do you have chest pain? If yes, go to 'I have chest pain – nobody hit me!' (p. 127)

• Do you have any allergies?

No. Could indicate serious head injury or metabolic disturbance – low blood sugar.
Close observation is necessary – Do not leave the player alone!

Observe
Use your instincts!
Does the player look very sick? Are they pale, Sweaty, or Clammy?
If the player looks sick or you are unsure in any way, seek medical assistance immediately.

Here are a few things to observe for

Airway

Look in the player's mouth and make sure nothing is blocking the airway. Remove anything in the mouth and make sure the player can breathe.

A player may complain of feeling their airway close in. This may be due to an anaphylactic reaction so enquire about allergies or any bites. See Anaphylaxis on p. 43.
See Chapter 5 for further information.

Breathing

Has the player difficulty breathing? Is the player asthmatic?
Watch the movement of the chest and feel the rib cage moving in and out equally on both sides. If this is not happening or the player is in great distress, go to the ABC chapter (p. 21).

Circulation

Feel for the player's pulse. The best pulse to feel is the carotid pulse in the neck (Fig. 6.1).

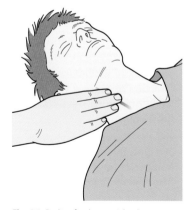

Fig. 6.1 Feeling for the carotid pulse.

Level of consciousness

Check if the player is alert by observing them. Are their eyes open?
Do they seem very sleepy?
If they are drifting in and out of consciousness, talk to them and keep them awake.

A player may have lost consciousness briefly as a result of a faint (see Faint, p. 43)
Seek immediate medical attention and urgent transfer to hospital.

Eye movement
Stand in front of the player and ask them to look at you.

- Watch to see if they can focus their eyes on you

- If their eyes are rolling in their head or unable to stay in one spot, this may indicate a head injury or concussion

- Ask them to follow your finger as you draw out an imaginary 'H' in front of them

- Observe to ensure that the eyes follow in all directions

- Any lack of movement in one direction or blurred vision when doing this suggests a head injury

- Tell the player to cover one eye with their hand. Hold up a number of fingers and ask 'How many fingers do you see?'

INFORMATION

Feeling for a player's pulse

You can feel the pulse by running the first two fingers of your right hand (index and middle finger) alongside the outer edge of your trachea (windpipe). Press your fingers in and move them outwards about two finger breadths – you should be able to feel the pulsation of the artery. It is sometime difficult to feel in a heavy person, so you may have to press a bit deeper. Since the carotid arteries supply a lot of the blood to the brain, it's important not to press on both of them at the same time!

If **the person has no pulse**, check the other side. Look at the colour of the player. A person with no pulse will be unconscious and very pale; go immediately to the ABC chapter (p. ••) (check airway and breathing), start chest compressions and **transfer to hospital as soon as possible.**

A person exercising is likely to have a fast pulse! What is most worrying is a very slow or absent pulse or a pulse that doesn't slow down when exercise has ceased. Seek medical assistance in these cases.

- The wrong answer a number of times suggests a head injury

Verbal response
Ask the player the following questions.

- 'What day is it?' (Time)

- 'What's your name?' (Person)

- 'Where are you?' (Place)

Incorrect answers or confused babble indicate a serious problem. The player must be observed closely and assessed by trained medical personnel urgently.

Movement

• Watch the way the player is lying or sitting. Are they moving all their limbs normally?

• Ask them to touch your finger and then touch their nose. Repeat this task, moving your finger in a few directions and observe for coordination. Lack of coordination may indicate a head injury. Go to Chapter 11 and transfer to hospital

Rule out serious injury

• At any stage if the player becomes unconscious go to the ABC chapter (p. 21)

• Any collapse is potentially life-threatening

• If the patient is complaining of neck or back pain, go to Chapter 7

• Transfer straight to hospital if in any doubt!

 INFORMATION

Things to check for

• Dehydration
   • Heat stroke
   • Hypothermia
   • Allergic reaction (anaphylaxis)
   • Diabetes

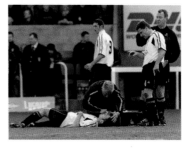

Dehydration

Dehydration involves the loss of water and important blood salts. **It may occur in any sport** but is more common in endurance sports (marathon running, triathlons, cross-country skiing). Usually occurs at high altitudes and in extremes of temperature – very hot or very cold.

What do I check for?

• The player will be extremely thirsty

• Ask them to open their mouth!

• They will have very dry lips and a dry mouth

• They may also have a fast pulse

• The player's urine will be extremely concentrated – very, very yellow

Signs of serious dehydration

• Blue lips

• A weak pulse

- Quick breathing
- Confusion

See 'What should I do?' for dehydration (p. 42).

Hyperthermia (heat stroke)

Feel the player's forehead with the back of your hand. Are they extremely hot or cold? (Compare with your own forehead if in doubt.)

What should I check for?

- Mental confusion
- Muscle cramps
- Headaches
- Nausea and vomiting
- Extremely warm
- Absence of sweating

See 'What should I do?' for hyperthermia (p. 44).

Hypothermia (very cold)

What should I check for?

- Shivering – becomes more severe and uncontrollable the colder the player gets
- Goose bumps
- Quick and shallow breathing
- Confusion
- Blue lips, ears, fingers and toes

See 'What should I do?' for hypothermia (p. 45).

Allergic reaction (anaphylaxis)

Anaphylaxis is a sudden, severe and potentially fatal allergic reaction that can involve any part of the body (such as skin, the airway and the heart). The symptoms may occur in minutes to hours after contact with the allergic substance.

Common causes

- Food
- Medication
- Insect bites
- Exercise

What will the player complain of?

- Light-headedness/dizziness
- Tingling sensation
- Itching
- Metallic taste in the mouth
- Hives
- Warmth
- Asthma
- Swelling of the mouth and/or throat area
- Difficulty breathing
- Loss of consciousness

It is important to act quickly if anaphylaxis is suspected. See 'What should I do?' for anaphylaxis (p. 43).

Diabetes – insulin reaction (hypoglycaemia)

This occurs when there is too much insulin in the body, which causes the blood sugar level to drop. In a diabetic person it may be caused by taking too much medication, by failing to eat, by heavy exercise and by emotional factors.

What should I check for?

- Fast breathing
- Dizziness
- Weakness
- Change in level of consciousness
- Problems with vision
- Sweating
- Headaches
- Numb hands or feet
- Hunger

Diabetic coma

In this condition there is too much sugar and too little insulin. In diabetic people, it is caused by eating too much sugar, by not taking medications, and by stress and infection. It is unlikely to occur during a game but it is important to be aware of the signs.

What should I check for?

The signs develop more slowly than with an insulin reaction, sometimes over days.

- Drowsiness
- Confusion
- Deep and fast breathing
- Thirst
- Dehydration
- Fever
- Change in consciousness
- Peculiar sweet or fruity smelling breath

See 'What should I do?' for diabetes (p. 44).

Faint

A faint is a temporary loss of consciousness as a result of reduction in blood flow to the brain. This may be caused by vigorous exercise or dehydration following sports.

After fainting a player should return to normal fairly quickly. If the player still has weakness or an inability to speak it may be more than a simple faint and they should be transferred to hospital immediately.

See 'What should I do?' for faint (p. 43).

Cramps or other orthopaedic condition

A muscle cramp or bony injury may be a cause of collapse. These injuries are normally not life-threatening and are dealt with in individual chapters depending on the site of the injury.

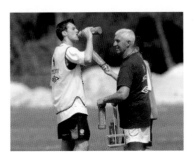

WHAT SHOULD I DO?

It is very important to make sure the airway is open at all times. See the ABC chapter (p. ●●).

Talk to the player

- It is extremely important to talk to a collapsed player
- Reassure them that they are going to be looked after
- Explain what you are doing
- Any drop in consciousness may indicate a serious event. Go to the ABC chapter (p. ●●) immediately!

Remove safely from the field of play

A collapsed, unconscious player should be regarded as having a neck injury until proved otherwise. Full spinal precautions are necessary for transfer. See Chapter 7.

A collapsed player with no neck or back injury should be removed to the sidelines with the assistance of one individual on each side and placed in a safe, dry area on their back with support for their neck.

Emergency transfer to hospital

- Any unconscious player or player in the **Red Zone** should be transferred to hospital immediately. **Continue to treat as per ABC chapter**

Avoid further injury

- No player who has had a collapse without trauma should be allowed to return to play unless assessed by trained personnel

 INFORMATION

Remember the Three Rs

- **R**ecognize symptoms
- **R**eact quickly
- **R**eview what happened – be sure to prevent it from occurring again.

Rehydration

The treatment of dehydration is to replace lost fluids.

- For exercise-related dehydration, cool water is best
- Sports drinks with electrolytes are also helpful
- Place the player in a cool sheltered area

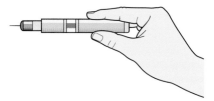

Fig. 6.2 Injectable adrenaline (epinephrine) EpiPen®.

- Tell the player to sip the water slowly until thirst is quenched
- Observe closely until they show signs of improvement
- In extremes of dehydration, the player may require intravenous fluids. This decision should be made by trained personnel. **Intravenous fluids should only be given under close observation**

Anaphylaxis

Act quickly! Seconds count!

- Seek medical assistance immediately
- Call for an ambulance. Tell them you have a player with an anaphylactic reaction. Tell them to bring adrenaline (ephinephrine)
- If a player has a known allergic reaction, antihistamine or asthma medications may be given
- Trained personnel may administer self-injectable adrenaline. Refer to the instructions that come with the pen for use

Faint

The aim of treatment is to get more oxygen to the brain. Falling to the floor will usually achieve this, as the head is then at the same level as the heart. If the player is supported while fainting and held upright, the blood will not go to the brain.

- Place the player on the ground with their feet raised above the level of their head
- If you are unable to lie the player on the ground, they should sit down with their head between their knees
- Observe the player closely until they feel normal
- Only allow them to stand up with assistance

If the fainting occurs only once it is normally not suspicious. However, if it occurs more frequently the player should seek medical attention.

Diabetes

Looking for the signs and symptoms will help distinguish the two diabetic emergencies. If the player is conscious, ask **two important questions** to figure out what the problem is.

- 'Have you eaten today?' Someone who has eaten but has not taken medication may be in a diabetic coma

- 'Have you taken your medication today?' Someone who has not eaten but has taken medication may be having an insulin reaction

Deciding between the two may be difficult! Of the two conditions, **insulin reaction** is the one that requires prompt action.

What should I do?

The player needs sugar, quickly! If conscious, give sugar in any form – sweets, fruit juices, sports drinks. Sugar given to a player with low blood sugar can be life-saving.

If the player is suffering from a diabetic coma, the sugar will *not* cause them harm.

If in doubt, give sugar!

Continue to monitor the player and transfer immediately to hospital.

INFORMATION

Always look for or ask about an identity bracelet that may reveal a player's condition.

Hyperthermia (heat stroke)

A player who has been in extremes of heat will need to cool down.

- Move the player to a cool area (indoors or at least in the shade)
- Remove sweaty clothes and dry off sweat
- Actively cool the player. Bathe in cool water. A hyperthermia vest may be applied
- Place a cool wet towel on the upper body, head, neck and groin
- A fan may be used
- Give plenty of water or sports drinks
- Observe closely – if temperature doesn't drop and the player is not coming around, transfer immediately to hospital

INFORMATION

Do not use ice or very cold water – this may cause hypothermia.

Hypothermia (low body temperature)

- Remove the athlete from play. Bring them indoors or to a warm sheltered area
- Remove wet clothes and replace them with dry ones
- Keep the player warm with towels, blankets, etc. (foil blanket or sleeping bag)
- Cover the player's head and neck to retain heat
- Make sure they are not dehydrated
- Give the player a warm, sweetened drink
- If the player is confused or there are changes in the mental status, transfer immediately to hospital

 INFORMATION

Do not use direct heat (such as hot water, a heating pad or a heat lamp) to warm a player.

Do not give the player alcohol or drinks containing caffeine.

COLLAPSE WITH TRAUMA

This topic is dealt with according to the site of the injury – see appropriate chapter.

Remember, **an unconscious player has a neck injury until proven otherwise**. Go to the ABC chapter (p. 21).

chapter 7

Player immobilization and transfer

M J Shelly, A R Poynton

Trained personnel should be responsible for head, neck and spine stabilization. These are the steps they should follow.

HEAD AND NECK STABILIZATION

How do I hold the head and neck steady?

Requirements

- Two people
- A hard cervical collar – a range of sizes or an adjustable one
- Sand bags
- Spinal board

Technique

- Kneel in a comfortable position above the player's head. Hands are placed on the side of the head or helmet, holding firmly (Fig. 7.1)
- Additional stability is achieved by resting your elbows on your thighs

- Fingers can be inserted into the ear holes of the helmet to ensure a good grip
- Reassure the athlete and tell them not to move
- If a hard collar is not available, continue to hold the head and neck steady until help arrives

Putting on a hard collar

Do not move the head and neck during the procedure.

How do I know which size?

- Ask your assistant to use their fingers to measure the distance from the base of the neck to the chin (Fig. 7.2). This gives you the size
- Identify which size collar best fits the neck (Fig. 7.3)

How do I put the collar on?

It is extremely important that the player's head does not move when you are putting on the hard collar.

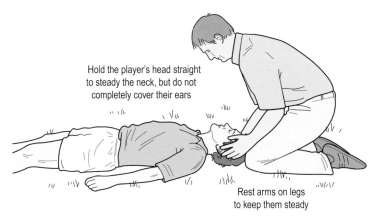

Hold the player's head straight to steady the neck, but do not completely cover their ears

Rest arms on legs to keep them steady

Fig. 7.1 Holding the head.

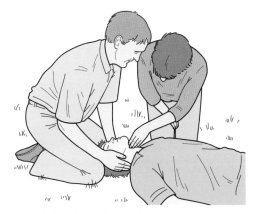

Fig. 7.2 How to measure the length of a player's neck.

While the head and neck are being held steady, the back of the collar should be slid behind the player's neck first and securely closed across the front (Figs 7.4, 7.5).

Remember, a hard collar alone does not properly secure the head and neck. **Continue to hold the head and neck steady until the player is transferred to a spinal board and their head is secured with sandbags and tape** (Fig. 7.6).

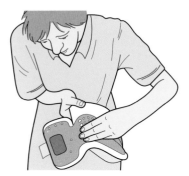

Fig. 7.3 Accurate sizing of the hard collar.

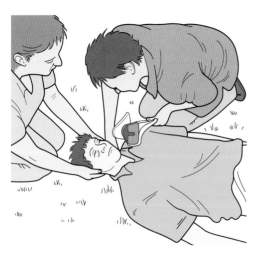

Fig. 7.4 Putting on the hard collar.

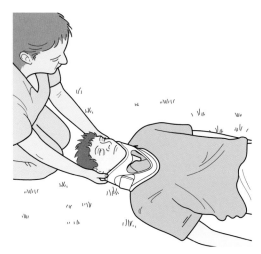

Fig. 7.5 The hard collar in place.

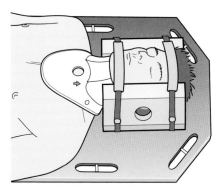

Fig. 7.6 Player's head and neck secure with sandbags and tape.

SPINE STABILIZATION – HOW TO LOGROLL

- **All directions** for movement must come from the team

doctor/suitably trained individual stationed at the player's head

- To safely perform a logroll, you will need **at least four**

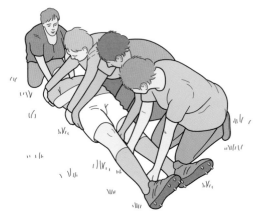

Fig. 7.7 Position for logrolling.

people – fewer than this number is unsafe and logrolling should not be attempted

- **The player must only be moved once – when being transferred to a spinal board**
- If the player is lying face down or has no pulse they will have to be logrolled onto their back to start CPR
- If an unconscious player with a possible spine injury vomits, they will have to be logrolled on to their side to avoid choking

Logroll with the player lying on their back

- The people who will logroll the player are placed along

one side of the player – at the chest, pelvis, and legs, in the kneeling position (Fig. 7.7)
- The spinal board is placed on the other side of the player
- **The person in charge (i.e. person holding the player's head and neck) gives the order to logroll the player**
- A good way to ensure everyone moves **at the same time** is to say 'ready to move, and move'
- The player's head, shoulders, chest, hips and legs are logrolled **at the same time** until the player is at right angles to the spinal board (Fig. 7.8)
- The spinal board is then slid under the player (see Fig. 7.8) and the player can be lowered

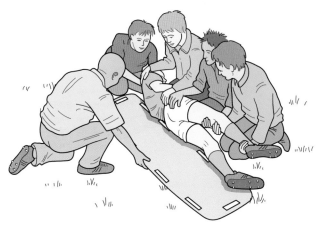

Fig. 7.8 Correct logrolling technique

onto the board, under the instructions of the person holding the head

- The person at the hips can reach for the spinal board if no one else is around to help
- The head or helmet should be secured to the spinal board with sandbags and tape (Fig. 7.6). **The player's head and neck are now secure**

Logroll with the player lying on their front

- The people involved in the logroll should assume the same positions as above except that the spinal board should be placed on the

same side as the people logrolling the player (i.e. they kneel on it to begin the logroll)

- **The person holding the athlete's head must use the crossed-arm technique.** This allows you to 'unwind' your arms as the player is logrolled
- **The person in charge (i.e. the person holding the player's head and neck) gives the order to logroll the player – 'ready to move, and move'**
- The player's head, shoulders, chest, hips and legs are logrolled **at the same time** until the player is at right angles to the spinal board

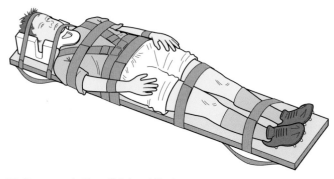

Fig. 7.9 Player on a spinal board fully immobilized.

- The player is then carefully lowered on to the spinal board to complete the logroll
- The player should be secured at chest, pelvis, thighs and ankles (Fig. 7.9)
- Remember – the player's neck is not safe until their head and neck are secured with sandbags and tape
- The player on the spinal board can now be placed, carefully, on a stretcher

TRANSFERRING A PLAYER

A player that is badly injured will need to be moved off the field on a stretcher (Fig. 7.10) **Ensure they have no neck or back injuries, or place on a spinal board (see above).**

1. Get the player to lie on their back
2. Help them to roll on to their good side
3. Support the injured limb if necessary
4. Place the stretcher underneath the raised half of their body
5. Gently lower the player down and move them into the middle of the stretcher
6. Five assistants are required for a proper stretcher lift: one assistant at each side of the hips and shoulders and one assistant at the head
7. When lifting, the leader should begin a countdown to ensure that the stretcher is lifted safely and evenly by all assistants – **'1, 2, 3, And Lift!'.**

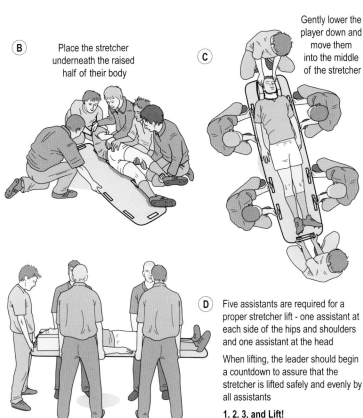

A A player who is badly injured will need to be moved off the field on a stretcher

Ensure they have no neck or back injuries

Get the player to lie on their back

Help them to roll on to their good side

Support the injured limb if necessary

B Place the stretcher underneath the raised half of their body

C Gently lower the player down and move them into the middle of the stretcher

D Five assistants are required for a proper stretcher lift - one assistant at each side of the hips and shoulders and one assistant at the head

When lifting, the leader should begin a countdown to assure that the stretcher is lifted safely and evenly by all assistants

1, 2, 3, and Lift!

Fig. 7.10 Transferring a player by stretcher.

Skin injury

A M Byrne, A Byrne

ABRASIONS AND LACERATIONS

Abrasions are shallow wounds where the top layers of skin are scraped off but the wound does not extend far beneath the surface of the skin. They are usually caused by falls on to a hard surface, scraping the hands, elbows and knees (Fig. 8.1).

Lacerations are deep cuts that may require stitches to heal properly. They occur when the skin is penetrated by a sharp object or when the skin is crushed against a bony edge, such as the cheekbone. Cuts that continue to bleed after 15 minutes of direct pressure, extend deep into the skin or have gaping edges may require stitches (Fig. 8.2) (**Red Zone injury**).

Treatment

- **Wear protective gloves**

Green zone

- **Remove all dirt and foreign material in the wound**

- **Wash with mild antiseptic creams and soap and warm water**
- **Use of antibacterial ointment is optional**
- **Apply dry adhesive dressing**
- **Return to play**

Amber Zone

- If difficulty bringing wound edges together, wound may need paper stitches and dressings
- Use ice pack to relieve immediate pain and swelling
- The player can return to play after appropriate treatment
- If the player has never had a tetanus injection or it is more than 10 years since his last injection, see doctor after play for treatment

Red Zone

- **Does the cut continue to bleed after 15 minutes of direct pressure?**
- **Is their foreign material that you can't remove in wound?**
- **Can muscle, tendons, blood vessels, nerves, or bone be seen at base of cut?**

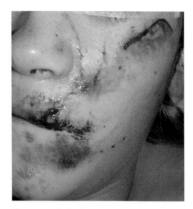

Fig. 8.1 Multiple abrasions and lacerations to the face following a fall on gravel. (Courtesy of Ms Eilis Fitzgerald.)

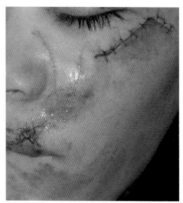

Fig. 8.2 Repair of lacerations with suturing, performed by a plastic surgeon. (Courtesy of Ms Eilis Fitzgerald.)

- **Any swelling, redness or pus in wound after a few days?**

See doctor immediately.

BLISTERS

Blisters, often thought to be minor injuries, can stop an athlete from continuing play. They form when the skin rubs against another surface, such as the heel rubbing against the back of a shoe, or the hand rubbing against a racket handle. The friction caused results in tearing in the upper layers of skin and fluid seeps into the torn area while the skin surface remains intact. Blisters are more likely to form on moist skin and in warm conditions.

Prevention

- Use of petroleum jelly or talcum powder to reduce friction
- Wear correct size shoes
- Wear appropriate socks
- Consider the use of 'second skin', methylated spirits rubbed on with cotton wool, potassium permanganate

Treatment

Green zone

- **Cover small, intact blisters with non-adhesive dressing**
- **Return to play**

Amber Zone

- If blister bursts, clean area with mild antiseptic soap and water

- Apply antiseptic ointment
- Cover with dry, non-adhesive dressing
- Return to play
- Avoid weightbearing training where possible

Red Zone

- **Large, painful blisters need treatment to stop the blister enlarging and avoid infection**
- **See doctor to drain large, intact blisters**
- **See doctor for treatment of infected blisters that are red, swollen and oozing pus**
- **May need antibiotics**

SUNBURN

Prevention

- Sunburn prevention is essential for all outdoor sporting events
- Use a sunscreen SPF 15 or higher
- Apply 20–30 minutes before sun exposure and regularly during exposure
- Wear a wide-brimmed hat when possible
- Ultraviolet-protective clothing is now available for children and adults

Treatment

Green zone

- **Mild sunburn can be treated with after-sun lotion**

- **Protect the affected area with clothing/hat**
- **Avoid further sunburn with SPF lotion**

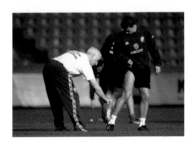

Amber Zone

- For moderate sunburn, stay out of direct sunlight
- Encourage gentle rehydration with sips of water
- Place cold, damp towel over affected area
- Cool bath for 10 minutes
- After-sun lotion or calamine lotion to area
- If no skin blistering, consider a 1% hydrocortisone lotion for symptom relief, or flamazine

Red Zone

- **If severe burn with blistering, cover blistered area with non-adhesive dressing**
- **Paracetamol for pain control**
- **See doctor if blisters continue to ooze or any pus at blister sites**

chapter 9

Strains, sprains and tears

J Walsh, S J Eustace

Muscle, tendon and ligament strains, sprains and tears are the most common group of all the injuries occurring in sport. The majority of these injuries are relatively minor. However, it is important to recognize the serious injuries early to allow for immediate treatment.

Muscle

Muscles (Fig. 9.1) are composed of an upper (origin), middle (body) and lower section (insertion). Muscle injuries are usually caused by overstretching the muscle during sudden acceleration/deceleration (strain/tear) or from a direct blow to the muscle (bruise/contusion). The most commonly injured muscles are the hamstrings, the quadriceps (thigh) and the calf muscles.

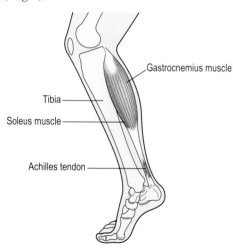

Fig. 9.1 Muscle and tendon.

Tendon

Tendons (Fig. 9.1) are thick bands of fibrous tissue that attach muscles to bones. Tears to tendons are most likely to occur at the junction of the muscle with the tendon and usually occur without warning (typically in older athletes). The most commonly injured areas are at the ankle (Achilles tendon), thigh (quadriceps tendon), biceps and the shoulder (supraspinatus tendon).

Ligament

Ligaments (Fig. 9.2) are thick fibrous bands attaching bone to bone in moving joints. They help to stabilize joints during movement. Ligament injuries typically occur during sudden movements (especially twisting) of the joint involved and most frequently occur in the knee, ankle, shoulder, elbow and fingers.

Red Zone

- **Complete muscle rupture**
- **Complete tendon rupture**
- **Complete ligament rupture**

Amber Zone

- **Significant bruising (e.g. 'Dead leg')**
- **Incomplete tear to muscle**

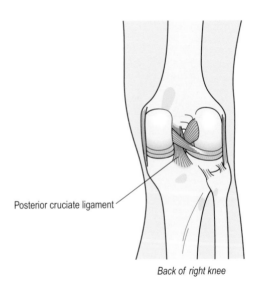

Posterior cruciate ligament

Back of right knee

Fig. 9.2 Ligament.

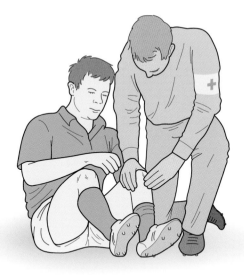

Fig. 9.3 Mild knee strain following a tackle. Once the injury is assessed and the player can perform the necessary skills, they may return to competition immediately.

- Incomplete tendon tear
- Incomplete ligament tear

Green zone

- **Muscle soreness**
- **Muscle cramp**
- **Minor bruising**
- **Mild tenderness over tendon (mild tendon strain)**
- **Mild tenderness over joint line (mild ligament strain)**

What should I do?

Speak to the player

- 'What happened?'
- 'Where does it hurt?'
- 'What kind of pain is it?'
- 'Did you feel/hear a crack/snap?'
- 'Does it feel like you have pulled a muscle?'

Problem identification

- Get player to point to sore area

Observe

- Look at the affected area for signs of swelling/redness/deformity
- Compare the affected area with the other side: Is there a difference?

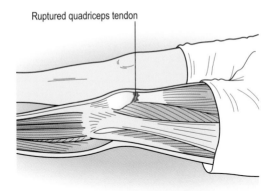

Ruptured quadriceps tendon

Fig. 9.4 Complete quadriceps rupture. Red Zone – Transfer immediately to hospital.

Rule out serious injury

- Ask the player to move the injured area on their own
- Does this cause pain?
- Does the injured area appear deformed? **You must be aware of the possibility of an underlying fracture/complete tear requiring hospital transfer (Red Zone Injury)**

Touch

- Touch the area to feel for warmth (indicates inflammation)
- Touching allows you to assess the extent of the pain
- Is there a specific point of tenderness?
- Does gentle movement of the joint cause pain? (Move the joint throughout its pain-free range of motion)
- Ask the player to move the joint themselves. If they can't move the area without severe pain, the injury almost certainly falls into the red zone **(Red Zone Injury)**

Skills assessment

- Ask the player to stand and move the injured area in the same way they would while competing. For instance:
  - with a lower limb injury, is the player able to stand unaided on the affected leg? (Getting the player to hop in a circle is a useful test for the lower limb)
  - with an upper limb injury, can the player move their

arm throughout its full range of motion, grip, push and pull against a heavy object?

What should I check for?

Talk to the player

- Does the player think they can continue? ('Yes' may actually mean 'No' in this situation)
- Reassure the player and explain what you are doing and why

Remove from the field of play

- Minor injuries (Green Zone) may be dealt with on the pitch
- Removing the player allows you to reassess the situation and make a less pressured and more informed decision on the sideline
- When an injury is identified, assess whether it is safe to remove the player from the pitch without additional splinting or assistance
- **Do not remove a player from the pitch unless it is safe to do so**

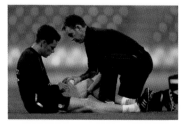

Emergency transfer

- Does the injury require urgent medical attention? Consider this if you suspect an underlying fracture/the player has an open wound (**Red Zone Injury**)
- If you suspect a complete tear of the muscle/tendon/ligament (**Red Zone Injury**), do not move the player from the pitch until you have enough personnel to do so without unnecessarily moving the injured area
- If you suspect a fracture (**Red Zone Injury**), manage the player as if there was a definite fracture

Avoid further injury

Green zone

- **Observe the player when they return to play, they may be unable to 'run off' the injury**
- **If they are still showing obvious signs of discomfort after 5 minutes, the injury is unlikely to resolve without further treatment. The player should be substituted and the injury reassessed**

Amber Zone

- **Be aware that partial tears (especially in ligaments) will usually, but not always, result in pain on movement of the affected area with or without swelling and tenderness**

- Athletes frequently feel able to return to the field of play immediately following a partial tear, resulting in more severe injury and possible complete tear of the muscle/tendon/ligament

Red Zone

- **Do not delay in transferring the patient with a suspected/obvious complete tear or fracture. Under no circumstances should these injuries wait until the game has finished**

Treatment

- See boxes on
  - Rest, ice, compression, elevation, diagnosis (RICED)
  - Putting on a splint

and the section on transferring a player in Chapter 7.

Muscle

What should I check for?

- Usually caused by collision with another player
- Muscle body will be warm, swollen and diffusely tender over the general area
- Stretching the muscle produces severe pain in the affected area
- There may be muscle (Fig. 9.4) deformity, or a palpable defect

and there will be a marked decrease in muscle strength and movement

- The player will be unable to perform a Skills assessment

What should I do?

- Remove the player from the pitch (**RICE**) and splint the injury
- Transfer to medical centre for further assessment and treatment

Tendon

What should I check for?

- Usually happens during sudden acceleration/deceleration
- Specific area of tenderness over affected tendon, with local swelling
- The player may have heard/felt a 'snapping' sensation when the injury occurred
- The player will be unable to perform a **S**kills assessment

What should I do?

- Remove from pitch (**RICE**) and splint the injury
- Transfer to a medical centre for further assessment and treatment

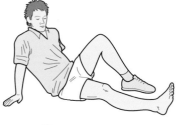

Rest
- Stop the activity
- Avoid as much movement as possible
- Don't put any weight on the injured part

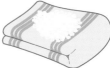

Ice
- Reduces pain, swelling and bleeding
- Hold the ice pack firmly in place with a bandage
- Don't put directly on bare skin

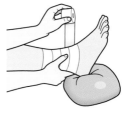

Compression
- Firm bandaging helps to reduce the bleeding and swelling

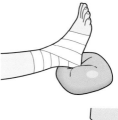

Elevation
- Helps to stop the bleeding and reduce swelling
- Keep the injured part raised as much as possible

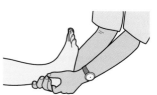

Diagnosis
- Consult trained personnel if you are worried about your injury, or if the pain or swelling gets worse

Fig. 9.5 RICED.

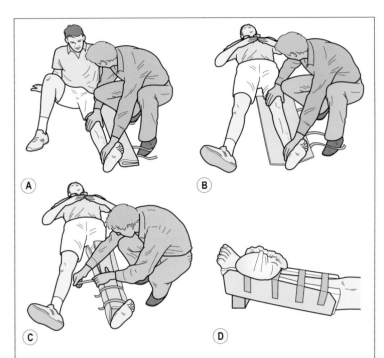

Steps

1. Place the splinting material along the underside of the leg so that it extends from above the underside of the knee to below the heel **(A)**.
2. Lift the leg, making sure to hold above and below the injured area to prevent movement.
3. Slip the splint underneath the leg and lay the leg gently on top of the splint **(B)**.
4. Fold the splinting material up around the sides of the leg.
5. Tie the splinting material into place below and above the fracture **(C)**.
6. The splint should be tight enough so the player cannot move the leg.
7. Apply ice to the injured area and keep it elevated **(D)**.
8. Transfer the patient by stretcher to the ambulance (see Ch. 7).

Warning: Don't tie the splint on too tightly. This could impede the circulation.

This information is not intended to be a substitute for professional medical advice and treatment.

Fig. 9.6 Putting on a splint.

Ligament

What should I check for?

- Usually happens when player is tackled/twists awkwardly (Fig. 9.7)
- Area of marked tenderness over the affected joint line – there may be associated joint swelling
- There will be instability of the joint on examination and pain on stressing the ligament will be a prominent feature
- The player will be unable to perform a **S**kills assessment

What should I do?

- Remove from pitch (**RICE**) and splint the injury
- Transfer to medical centre for further assessment and treatment

Muscle

What should I check for?

- Usually caused by collision with another player
- Muscle body will be warm, swollen and diffusely tender over the general area
- Stretching the muscle produces moderate pain in the affected area
- There will be **no** muscle deformity; however, there will be a decrease in muscle strength with or without a decrease in movement
- The player will be unable to perform an adequate **S**kills assessment

What should I do?

- Player cannot return to play

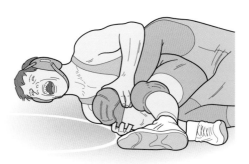

Fig. 9.7 A twisted knee scenario that may indicate ligament injury.

- Remove the player from the pitch (**RICE**)

Tendon

What should I check for?

- Usually happens during sudden acceleration/ deceleration
- Specific area of tenderness over affected tendon
- The player will be unable to perform an adequate **S**kills assessment

What should I do?

- Player cannot return to play
- Remove from pitch and reassess injury on sideline
- If you suspect a tear, **RICE**, splint the injury and seek medical advice following the game

Ligament

What should I check for?

- Usually happens when player is tackled/twists awkwardly
- Area of tenderness over the affected joint line – there may be associated joint swelling
- No instability of the joint on examination but pain will be a prominent feature
- The player will be unable to perform an adequate **S**kills assessment

What should I do?

- Player cannot return to play
- Remove from pitch and reassess injury on sideline
- If you suspect a tear, **RICE**, splint the injury and seek medical advice following the game

Muscle

What should I check for?

- Usually caused by collision with another player
- Muscle body will be warm, swollen and mildly tender over the general area
- Stretching the muscle produces mild pain in the affected area

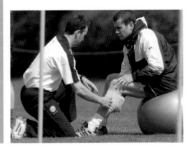

- There will be **no** muscle deformity, decrease in muscle strength or decrease in movement
- The **S**kills assessment will be normal

What should I do?

- Player can return to play (continue to observe)
- In the case of muscle cramp, treat with icing, massage and gentle stretching

Note: The exact underlying cause of cramp is unknown but it is thought to be partly due to dehydration and hypoglycaemia with or without an electrolyte imbalance.

Maintaining adequate hydration and the use of isotonic energy drinks may help to prevent this.

Tendon

What should I check for?

- Usually happens during sudden acceleration/deceleration
- Small but specific area of tenderness over affected tendon

- The **S**kills assessment will be normal

What should I do?

Player can return to play. (Observe closely – tendon strains can become tendon tears!)

Ligament

What should I check for?
(Fig. 9.3)

- Usually happens when player is tackled/twists awkwardly
- Area of tenderness over the affected joint line – no associated swelling
- No instability of the joint on examination
- The **S**kills assessment will be normal

What should I do?

- Player can return to play (Again observe closely – often, players have been allowed to play on with severe and even complete ligament tears)
- **If you have ANY suspicion that there is even a partial tear, substitute the player.**

chapter 10

Broken bones

J Walsh, P J Kenny

Broken bones occur commonly in contact sports. They can also occur in individual sports such as skiing, riding and gymnastics. There are many different methods that can be used to describe fractures but, for the purposes of this section, they have been divided into two types: closed and open fractures (Fig. 10.1).

INFORMATION

Closed

- The bone is fractured and may be markedly deformed; however the skin surrounding the broken bone remains intact

Open

- One or both of the broken bone ends pierces the skin
- The bone does not necessarily have to be visible for the fracture to be open (it may pierce the skin and return inside the body)

The on-field management of broken bones is divided into Red and Amber Zones. There are no green zone injuries in this section. All suspected fractures should be removed from the field of play.

Red Zone

- **Any open fracture**
- **Any long bone fracture**
- **Any fracture to a finger or toe with marked deformity**

Amber Zone

- **Broken finger or toe with minimal deformity**
- **Suspected fracture**

The majority of fractures will require immediate transfer to hospital. If in doubt, transfer!

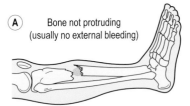

Ⓐ Bone not protruding (usually no external bleeding)

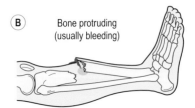

Ⓑ Bone protruding (usually bleeding)

Fig. 10.1 Open and closed fractures.

What should I check for?

Speak to the player

- 'What happened?'
- 'Where does it hurt?'
- 'What kind of pain is it?'
- 'Did you feel/hear a crack/ snap?'

Problem identification

- Get player to point to sore area

Observe

- Look at the affected area for signs of swelling/redness/ deformity
- Is the skin broken?
- Could this be an open fracture where the bone has gone back in?
- Compare the affected area with the other side – is there a difference?

Rule out serious injury

- Ask the player to move the injured area on their own
- Does this cause pain?
- Does the injured area appear deformed?

Touch for tenderness

- Touch the area to feel for warmth (indicates inflammation)
- Touching allows you to assess the extent of the pain

- Is there a specific point of tenderness?

Skills assessment

- Does gentle movement of the joint cause pain? (Move the joint throughout its full pain-free range of motion)
- Ask the player to move the joint themselves. Very few athletes will be able to perform any significant movement with an underlying fracture
- If you have a strong suspicion, or there is an obvious fracture, it is inappropriate to perform a skills assessment (**Red Zone Injury**). It may be clear from the sideline that the player will be unable to continue and that emergency treatment will be required
- If you suspect an underlying fracture the skills test will consist of moving the joint through its pain free range of motion and assessing whether the player can take any weight on the affected area

What should I do?

Talk to the player

Remove the player safely from the field of play

- If you suspect a fracture, the player is not going to be able to continue

- Stop play immediately. There is a potentially serious injury and the player may require urgent hospital treatment
- **Realigning the fracture (see box below) is the single most beneficial intervention that can be performed outside of a hospital environment**
- Realigning the bone will help to prevent compromise of the blood supply and the skin of the fractured area
- Realigning the bone will actually decrease the injured players' pain
- In the case of an open fracture, irrigate the area with sterile water and a sterile dressing before applying a splint
- Call for a stretcher from sideline (every sporting venue is required by law to have one)
- It is not always possible to realign a broken bone – if it is difficult to do so, put a splint on and prevent further movement of the bone ends

Emergency transfer to hospital

- Even if you only suspect a fracture, do not move the player from the pitch until you have enough personnel to do so without moving the injured area unnecessarily
- Splint the fracture (Figure 10.2, Page 73): This will provide stability to the realigned fracture and prevent further pain and damage due to unnecessary motion at the fracture site

Avoid further injury

- On the sideline, reassess the severity of the injury (do not remove a dressing from an open fracture unless necessary as this increases the risk of infection)
- Give analgesia (paracetamol and diclofenac) and fluids (except alcohol). Avoid food
- In the case of a well splinted, closed upper limb fracture, it is appropriate to transfer the player to hospital by car. Other long-bone closed fractures (humerus, tibia and fibula) should be transferred by ambulance wherever possible
- Open fractures, or any fracture where you suspect the local blood supply/skin has been compromised, should be transferred to hospital by ambulance

Treatment

The principles of management of Amber and Red Zone fractures are the same. If you are unsure which section a fracture falls into, treat it as a Red Zone injury.

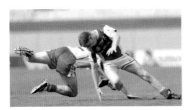

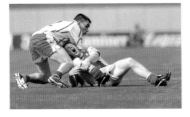

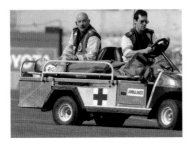

i INFORMATION

Realigning a broken leg

- Broken bones in the leg are serious injuries and are extremely painful
- They require immediate treatment by trained personnel
- The broken bones put a lot of pressure on the surrounding muscle and skin
- This may cut off the blood supply
- Any movement is not only painful but may worsen the injury
- If the bones are grossly out of position they can be realigned
- This process will relieve pain and should restore the blood supply.

Steps

1. Have another rescuer support the injured limb above the fracture site
2. Grasp the injured limb below the fracture site
3. Provide gentle traction – pull gently in line with the long axis of the bone
4. Move the lower part of the bone gently and carefully into line with the upper part
5. Release traction and splint the fracture.

Realignment of injuries to the upper limb is more difficult and should only be attempted by trained personnel. Place the injured arm in a splint to prevent movement of the bone ends.

Putting on a leg splint

Steps

1. Place the splinting material along the underside of the leg so that it extends from above the underside of the knee to below the heel (Fig. 10.2A)

2. Lift the leg, making sure to hold above and below the injured area to prevent movement

3. Slip the splint underneath the leg and lay the leg back gently on top of the splint (Fig. 10.2B)

4. Fold the splinting material up around the sides of the leg

5. Tie the splinting material into place below and above the fracture (Fig. 10.2C)

6. The splint should be tight enough so the player cannot move the leg

7. If the bone is protruding cover with a sterile gauze dressing (Fig. 10.2D)

8. Transfer the patient by stretcher to the ambulance (see Ch. 7).

This information is not intended to be a substitute for professional medical advice and treatment.

Think ahead

• To ensure the fracture is treated appropriately and quickly, ring ahead to the Emergency Department you are attending. This allows the necessary staff (orthopaedic team, radiologists, etc.) to be ready to review the injured player

• It is a good idea to be aware before you attend a game where the nearest emergency department is and how to get there. Some departments can only cater for minor injuries and will have to retransfer a player with a severe injury or open fracture. Knowing this will allow you to direct the injured player to the nearest appropriate facility and will avoid further distress and unnecessary delay in treating the fracture.

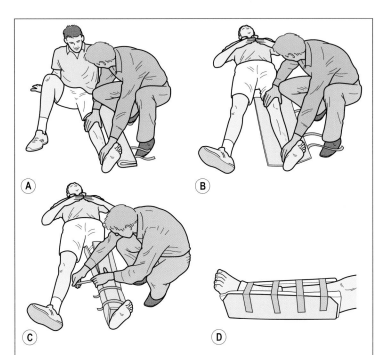

Steps

1. Place the splinting material along the underside of the leg so that it extends from above the underside of the knee to below the heel **(A)**.
2. Lift the leg, making sure to hold above and below the injured area to prevent movement.
3. Slip the splint underneath the leg and lay the leg gently on top of the splint **(B)**.
4. Fold the splinting material up around the sides of the leg.
5. Tie the splinting material into place below and above the fracture **(C)**.
6. The splint should be tight enough so the player cannot move the leg.
7. If the bone is protruding, cover with a sterile gauze dressing **(D)**.
8. Transfer the patient by stretcher to the ambulance (see Ch. 7).

   Warning: Don't tie the splint on too tightly. This could impede the circulation.

   This information is not intended to be a substitute for professional medical advice and treatment.

Fig. 10.2 Putting on a splint.

SECTION 3

Where is the Injury?

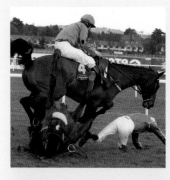

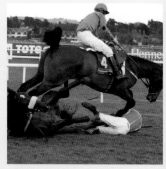

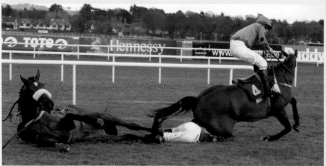

Head injuries

J S Butler, C Bolger

INTRODUCTION

Head injuries range from a simple blow to the head to serious injury causing brain damage and death. It is important to be able to deal with a simple concussion and recognize which head injuries are potentially serious.

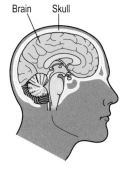

Fig. 11.1 Section through the skull and brain.

Brain   Skull

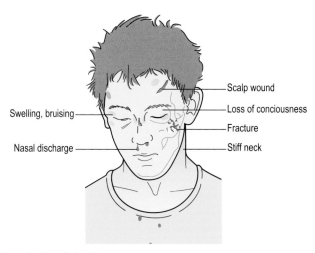

Scalp wound

Loss of conciousness

Fracture

Stiff neck

Swelling, bruising

Nasal discharge

Fig. 11.2 Indications of a head injury.

Red Zone

- **Unconscious athlete**
- **Severe head injury**
- **Skull fracture**
- **Seizure**

Amber Zone

- Concussion
- Scalp wound

Green zone

- **Minor blow to head (no concussion)**

If player is **unconscious** go to the ABC chapter (p. 21). **This is an emergency situation until proved otherwise.**

If the player is conscious do the following and **repeat this checklist regularly.**

What should I check for?

Speak to the player

- 'Are you OK?' 'Where did you get hit?' 'How did it happen?' 'Did you lose consciousness?'

Problem identification

- 'What's your name?' 'Where are you?' 'What's today's date?' 'Who are you playing?' 'What's the score?' A player who is unable to answer these questions is likely to be concussed

- 'Is your neck sore?' 'Have you a headache?' 'Are you dizzy or weak?' 'Do you feel sick?' 'Can you see properly?' 'Have you any weakness, pins and needles?' 'Can you move your hands and legs?'

The following symptoms indicate a **Red Zone injury** (emergency transfer to hospital).

- Headache
- Neck pain
- Tingling, pins and needles
- Vomiting
- Seizure
- Confusion
- Loss of memory – indicates concussion

Observe

- Look all around the face and skull for any bleeding (especially around eyes or behind ear) or scalp wounds
- Compare both sides of the skull
- Watch out for any depressed areas – skull fractures

Make sure the player is alert.

- Is the player opening their eyes?
- Can the player hold your gaze?

A player who cannot focus or whose eyes are rolling in their head suggests a serious injury

- Is there bruising around the eyes? – Serious head injury
- Are the pupils equal? – Unequal pupils indicate a serious injury
- Is the player shaking uncontrollably? – Go to Seizure section (p. 85)
- How is the player holding their neck? Is it straight or twisted?
- Are they moving all four limbs?
- Is there bruising or swelling of the face? – A serious face injury may also indicate a head injury
- Check the nose and ears to see if there is fluid or blood leaking out – Clear fluid indicates serious head injury

Rule out serious injury

- Look for signs of severe head injury, which are: intense headache, deteriorating level of responsiveness, drowsiness, nausea, vomiting, unequal pupil size, paralysis or loss of function of one side of body

(opposite head injury); paralysis or weakness on both sides may indicate a spinal injury (go to Chapter 7)

- Ask player to move arms and legs
- Check sensation of arms and legs

Touch (use gloves)

- Examine head and scalp for possibility of skull fracture
- Examine ears and nose for blood and cerebrospinal fluid leakage
- Examination of the eye: range of motion:
  - To check pupils, shine a pen torch into the eyes and check pupil response (Fig. 11.3)
  - If the pupil gets smaller, it is responding
  - Check both eyes
  - Next shine the light in the **right** eye and look at the **left** to see if it responds. Repeat the other side
  - Get player to follow your finger slowly with their eyes through an 'H' pattern (Fig. 11.4)

Skills assessment

If everything is normal at this stage, get the player to stand up, close their eyes and stand still; make sure the player is not falling to one side. If the player can walk and run on the spot

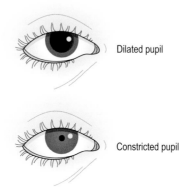

Dilated pupil

Constricted pupil

Fig. 11.3 Dilated pupil.

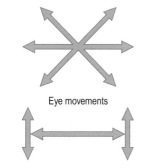

Eye movements

Fig. 11.4 Eye movements.

without difficulty, they can play on.

If there is no neck pain, check neck movements (Fig. 11.5):

- 'Touch your chin to your chest'
- 'Look up at the sky'
- 'Look over your left shoulder'
- 'Look over your right shoulder'
- 'Put your ear on your shoulder'

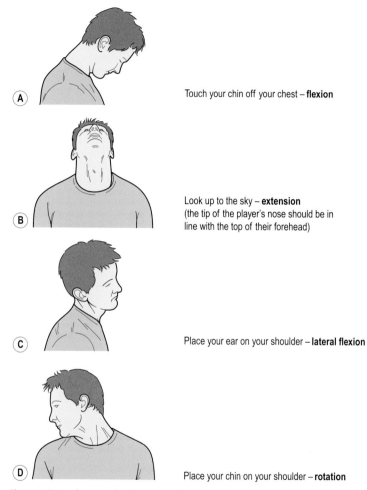

(A) Touch your chin off your chest – **flexion**

(B) Look up to the sky – **extension**
(the tip of the player's nose should be in
line with the top of their forehead)

(C) Place your ear on your shoulder – **lateral flexion**

(D) Place your chin on your shoulder – **rotation**

Fig. 11.5 Testing for range of neck movements.

What should I do?

Talk to the player

- Keep speaking to the player. The player may be disoriented. A quiet player who is not talking or responding is a worry

- Reassure the player – explain what you are doing and why

Remove from the pitch

- Do not remove a player from the pitch unless it is safe to do so

- When an injury is identified, assess whether it is safe to remove the player from the pitch without additional splinting or assistance

- Removing the player allows you to reassess the situation and make a less pressured and more informed decision on the sideline

- Minor injuries (**Green Zone**) may be dealt with on the pitch

- Reassure and explain what you are doing and why

Emergency transfer

- Any Red Zone injury should be transferred to hospital immediately

- If there is a suspicion of a neck injury, use neck and spine stabilization techniques (see Chapter 7)

Avoid further injury

- If there is any concern about a serious head injury or neck injury, only move the player if ABCs have been managed, and follow the neck injury guidelines technique to the letter

- A player with concussion should not play on. The Sports Concussion Assessment Tool (SCAT – Fig. 11.6) can be used

Treatment

- Any player who has suffered a head injury should be observed by a responsible person for 24 hours because, occasionally, there can be bleeding inside the skull several hours later

- Players should avoid alcohol or caffeine or any medication that may make them drowsy

Guidelines for return to play

It is recommended that a player should not return to competitive sport for 3 weeks.

In the first few days following a concussion, it is important to stress to the player that physical and mental rest is required.

Week 1

Days 1–3: No physical activity. Complete rest. If the player has

The SCAT Card (Sport Concussion Assessment Tool) Medical Evaluation

Name: _____   Date: _____

_____

Sport/Team: _____   Mouth guard? Y/N

1. SIGNS

Was there loss of conciousness/ unresponsiveness?   Y/N

Was there seizure or convulsive activity?   Y/N

Was there a balance problem/unsteadiness?   Y/N

2. MEMORY

Modified Maddocks questions (check if athlete answers correctly)

• At what venue are we? _____   Which half is it? _____   Who scored last? _____

• What team did we play last? _____   Did we win our last game? _____

3. SYMPTOM SCORE

Total number of positive symptoms (from reverse side of the card) _____

4. COGNITIVE ASSESSMENT (5 word recall)

	(examples)	Immediate	Delayed
Word 1 _____	cat	_____	_____
Word 2 _____	pen	_____	_____
Word 3 _____	shoe	_____	_____
Word 4 _____	book	_____	_____
Word 5 _____	car	_____	_____

Months in reverse order:

Jun-May-Apr-Mar-Feb-Jan-Dec-Nov-Oct-Sept-Aug-Jul

Digits backwards (check correct)

5-2-8	3-9-1	_____
6-2-9-4	4-3-7-1	_____
8-3-2-7-9	1-4-9-3-6	_____
7-3-9-1-4-2	5-1-8-4-6-8	_____

Ask delayed 5-word recall now.

5. NEUROLOGIC SCREENING

	Pass	Fail
Speech	_____	_____
Eye motion and pupils	_____	_____
Pronator drift	_____	_____
Gait analysis	_____	_____

Any neurologic screen abnormality necessitates formal neurological or hospital assessment

Fig. 11.6 SCAT card.

no problems, they can go on to the next stage

Days 4–7: Light aerobic activity – walking, jogging, cycling. No resistance training.

Week 2

- Sports-specific exercise
- Non-contact drills
- Skills, etc.

Week 3

- Full contact after medical clearance
- Return to competitive play
- The player should only move forward a stage if they are symptom-free
- If, at any point, the player complains of headaches, nausea, vomiting, double vision, they should seek medical assistance before return to play

SPECIFIC SPORTS EMERGENCIES

Red Zone – Straight to hospital

Amber Zone – Reassess

Green Zone – Responsible adult

Unconscious athlete

- Severe head injury – go to the ABC chapter (p. 21)

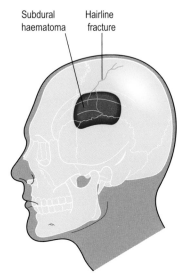

Subdural haematoma   Hairline fracture

Fig. 11.7 Skull fractures and haematomas.

Skull fracture (Fig. 11.7)

What should I check for?

The player will be in a lot of discomfort. Intense headache, deteriorating level of responsiveness, drowsiness, nausea, vomiting, unequal pupil size, paralysis or loss of function of one side of body. Examine the skull for a depression.

What should I do?

- Urgent transfer to hospital
- **Call ambulance**
- If conscious, support and reassure athlete, stabilizing

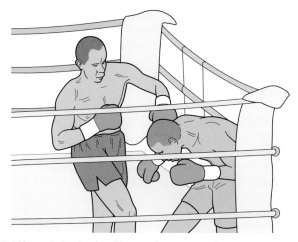

Fig. 11.8 A blow to the head such as this can easily cause concussion.

head and neck as per ABC guidelines (see Chapter 7)

- Apply pressure to bleeding scalp wound – not too hard if there is a skull depression

Concussion

A concussion is a violent jarring or shaking that results in a disturbance of brain function (Figs 11.8, 11.9). The player is normally disoriented – does not know where they are, does not know what the score is, etc.

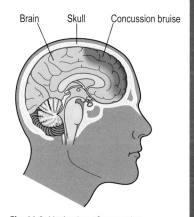

Brain   Skull   Concussion bruise

Fig. 11.9 Mechanism of concussion.

- Check the pupils are equal (see Fig. 11.4)
- Check for skull fractures
- Ensure no bleeding from nose or ears and check for facial bone injuries

- Dizziness or nausea (on recovery)
- Loss of memory (events immediately preceding injury or at time of injury)
- Mild generalized headache

What should I do?

- Remove the player from the pitch
- **Do not** allow the athlete to return to play
- Check level of consciousness and monitor vital signs until full recovery
- Place in the care of a responsible person. **Do not leave the player alone**
- Even if normal, advise the athlete to attend hospital if they develop headache, nausea, vomiting, excessive sleepiness
- If not normal, send to hospital immediately

When in doubt, sit them out!

Seizure

What should I check for?

A seizure is a sudden release of electrical activity from the brain resulting in altered behaviour or activity (Fig. 11.10).

- Observe: the player may complain of a 'funny' sensation before a seizure. Strange smells, visual disturbance – aura
- Tonic/clonic phase – sudden jerking movements of body which can last several minutes. Go to the ABC chapter (p. 21)
- The player may become unconscious
- May be accompanied by incontinence
- Tiredness and mild headache (on recovery)

What should I do?

- Make sure the player is safe and remove any nearby objects likely to result in injury
- Do not put anything in the player's mouth; they will not swallow their tongue

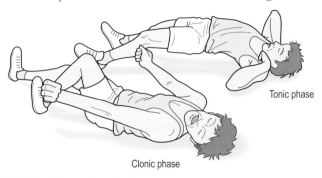

Tonic phase

Clonic phase

Fig. 11.10 Tonic and clonic phases of a seizure.

- Check the time that the seizure starts. Monitor duration if it lasts. Try to remember what movements the body makes
- Do not attempt to hold the player still: you cannot stop a seizure
- Loosen clothes around neck if necessary
- Remain calm and reassure the player after the seizure. Turn into the recovery position after the seizure while drowsy
- Immediate transfer to hospital
- A doctor or trained personnel may give rectal diazepam

Concussion

When can a player return to play after a concussion?

- No concussed player should return to training or play for a period of 3 weeks
- After 3 weeks they may only resume play when they are symptom-free and have medical clearance
- Coaches should seek medical clearance before permitting a player to take part in training or play. See Guidelines for return to play following concussion, below

i INFORMATION

Guidelines for return to play following concussion

Concussion is a 'trauma-induced alteration in mental status that may or may not involve loss of consciousness'. Most guidelines incorporate the following:

- If any symptoms are present during play or on static testing, the player should not continue
- If there is evidence of loss of consciousness, or post-concussive symptoms that persist beyond 20 minutes after the injury, no further participation should take place that day and the player should be referred for further assessment
- If an athlete sustains mild concussion that is fully resolved within 15–20 minutes, there is no evidence of loss of consciousness and the athlete finds that resuming activity does not cause any further symptoms, continued participation is permitted
- All the above scenarios require regular history-taking and physical examination and constant re-evaluation. If in doubt, refer for specialist medical review

Scalp injuries

What should I check for?

The scalp may bleed a lot, making a usually minor wound appear far worse. However, a scalp wound (Fig. 11.11) may be

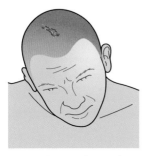

Fig. 11.11 An obvious scalp wound.

part of a more serious underlying head injury, such as a skull fracture, or may be associated with a neck/spinal injury, so careful assessment of the athlete for evidence of a serious head injury is essential.

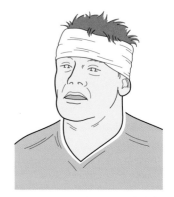

Fig. 11.12 A pressure bandage applied after treatment of a laceration.

What should I do?

Speak to the player:

- 'What's your name?'
- 'Where are you?'
- 'What day is today?'
- 'Do you have a headache?'
- 'Do you have double vision?'

Touch (use gloves):

- Check response of pupils to light (see Fig. 11.3)
- Check eye movements (see Fig. 11.4)
- Cover wound with sterile dressing or clean pad
- Apply firm direct pressure on pad

- Secure dressing with roller bandage

Following treatment of an uncomplicated laceration, a pressure bandage can be applied (Fig. 11.12) and the player may continue to participate, if they have no concussion. They should be assessed by trained personnel after the match.

What the doctor does

- **Uncomplicated scalp laceration** – can be approximated using a suture, skin stapler or skin glue
- **Children's scalp laceration** – can occasionally be approximated by tying the hair on either side.

chapter 12

Facial injuries

J S Butler, F Coffey, F Kearns

INTRODUCTION

Facial injuries are common in sport, particularly in contact sports. Typical injuries range from simple cuts and mild abrasions to a facial bone injury or broken jaw, with possible life-threatening airway problems. It is important to remember that there can be an associated head and neck injury.

This chapter is divided into four parts:

- Facial bones: nose and cheek bones
- Eyes and ears
- Jaw and mouth
- Cuts to the face

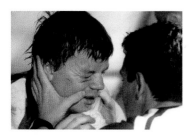

FACIAL BONES: NOSE AND CHEEK BONES

What should I check for?

Speak to the player

- 'Are you OK?' 'Where were you hit?'
- 'Where is the pain?' 'Did you hear a crack?'
- 'Do you feel any numbness on your face'
- 'Do you have difficulty breathing?'
- 'Can you see me OK?' (blurring/double vision)

Problem identification

- A 'crack' usually indicates a broken bone
- Numbness usually indicates a compressed nerve
- Visual disturbance may indicate an eye socket fracture or an injury to the eye itself
- Facial fractures may cause airway compromise and affect breathing

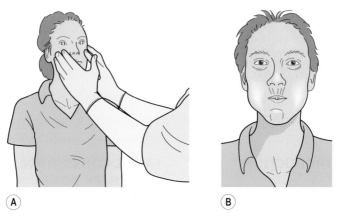

Fig. 12.1 Checking facial bones. **A.** Assessing for a eye socket fracture. **B.** Blow out your cheeks!

Observe

- Is there swelling/redness/ deformity/bloodshot eye/ abrasion/laceration?
- Compare the injured area with the uninjured side:
  - Is there asymmetry of the face? Asymmetry normally indicates swelling or a fracture
  - Is the nose displaced or the cheekbone depressed?

Rule out serious injury

- Is there a head injury?
- Injury of the spine?
- If worried about either of these, go to the relevant chapter

Touch (use gloves)

- Feel gently around facial bones for tenderness or a step (possible bone injury or break)
- Feel gently around the rim of the eye socket for tenderness or a step (possible broken bone) (Fig. 12.1A)
- Get the player to clench their teeth, assessing for malalignment (this might include a palate fracture)
- Place your finger and thumb in the player's mouth, holding on to the upper jaw. Assess whether the jaw is stable on gentle movement

Skills assessment

- Ask the player to blow out their cheeks, smile, whistle and wrinkle their forehead (Fig. 12.1B). If not normal, the player needs specialist review

What should I do?

Talk to the player

- Reassure and explain what you are doing and why

Remove from the pitch

- **Do not** remove a player from the pitch unless it is safe to do so
- Minor injuries (Green zone) may be dealt with on the pitch
- Removing the player allows you to reassess the situation and make a less pressured and more informed decision on the sideline
- When an injury is identified, assess whether it is safe to remove the player from the pitch without additional splinting or assistance

Emergency management

- ABC emergency management
- Emergency transfer to hospital if serious injury is suspected
- Occasionally a player with broken facial bones will insist on sitting up and leaning forward to get their breath

Avoid further injury

- Get the player off the field of play for further assessment/ management

- A player must not play on with a broken nose or cheekbone

Treat the problem

Nosebleed

Do not let the head tilt back.

- Ask the player to sit down. Tilt the head forwards to allow the blood to drain from the nostrils
- Put on gloves. Apply pressure to the fleshy part of the nose (not the bridge of the nose) using a clean gauze or tissue (Fig. 12.2)
- Most bleeding should stop within 10–15 minutes
- If bleeding stops and restarts, tell the player to reapply pressure
- If the bleeding lasts more than 30 minutes, **send the player to hospital**
- A **doctor** or other trained person may insert a nasal tampon dipped in adrenaline (epinephrine)

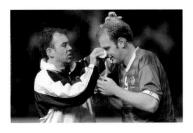

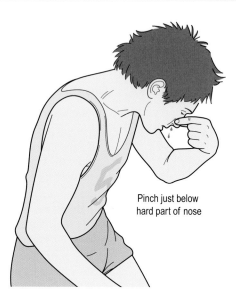

Pinch just below
hard part of nose

Fig. 12.2 Treating a nosebleed.

Broken nose

- The nose will appear crooked or asymmetrical (Fig. 12.3)
- Ask the player if they have broken their nose before. The crooked position may be normal
- Place a cold compress on the nose
- A **doctor** or trained person may try to correct the deformity. Explain to the player that this may be painful
- Place your thumb and index finger of your left hand on the bridge of the nose

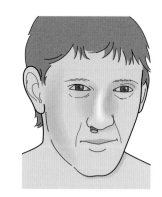

Fig. 12.3 Broken nose with nasal tampon in place.

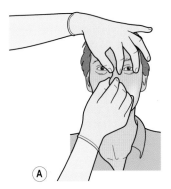 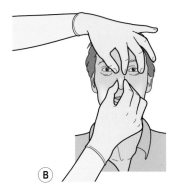

Fig. 12.4 Straightening a broken nose.

- Hold the nose with your index finger and thumb on the other hand
- Move the nose towards the midline (Fig. 12.4). This may require some force
- The player will often describe a 'click' or 'clunk'
- Observe the nose to assess straightness. If straight, apply tape to hold the nose in place
- If it is very difficult to correct, the player may need an anaesthetic. **Send to hospital**
- The player should be assessed by a doctor to make sure that the septum in between the nostrils is not deviated. If it is still deviated following correction, the player should go to hospital

Broken cheekbones

- If there are any fractures of the cheekbones or face, place a cold compress over the area
- Apply pressure to any cuts or lacerations with a sterile gauze
- **Send the player to hospital immediately**

EYES AND EARS

Eyes

Red Zone

- **Broken eye socket**
- **Eyelid laceration**
- **Damaged eyeball**
- **Loss of vision**

Amber Zone

- **Foreign body (unremovable)**
- **Double vision**

Green zone

- **Foreign body (removable)**
- **Lost contact lens**
- **Skin bruising around eye**

What should I check for?

Speak to the player

- 'Are you OK?' 'Where did you get hit?' 'How did it happen?'
- 'Can you see me?' 'Is your vision blurred?' 'Do you have double vision?'
- 'Do you feel anything in your eye?'
- 'Do you wear glasses or contact lenses?'

Problem identification

- Is there a foreign body in the eye?
- Is there anything floating in eye?
- Is there an injury to the eyeball or bruising of the skin around the eye (black eye)?
- Is there extreme pain?

Observe

- Is the injured eye different from the uninjured eye?

Rule out serious injury

- Is there a head injury?
- Is there a neck injury?
- Are the bones in the face broken?
- Is the eyeball damaged or is it 'just a black eye'?

Touch (use gloves)

- Examine pupils and eye movement:
- Shine a pen torch in the eyes to see if the pupils react

appropriately to light by getting smaller (constricting) (see Fig. 11.3, Ch. 11)

- Letter H sign (see Fig. 11.4, Ch. 11)
- Examine the rim of the eye socket for tenderness or a step – there may be a fracture
- Look at the eyeball and inspect pupil
- Cover uninjured eye and ask the player if they can see properly with the injured eye

Skills assessment

- If vision is normal at this stage and there is no pain, the player may return to play

What should I do?

Talk to the player

- Reassure and explain what you are doing and why

Remove from the pitch

- **Do not** remove a player from the pitch unless it is safe to do so
- Minor injuries (Green Zone) may be dealt with on the pitch
- Removing the player allows you to reassess the situation and make a less pressured and more informed decision on the sideline
- When an injury is identified, assess whether it is safe to remove the player from the pitch

Emergency management

- ABC emergency management
- Emergency transfer to hospital if serious injury is suspected

Avoid further injury

- Get the player to hold their head still to allow examination of the eye
- Do not rub or poke at the eye!

Treat the problem (put on gloves)

- Foreign bodies, including contact lenses, should be removed from the eye. This may be done by pouring sterile water over the eye (Fig. 12.5)
- Cover eye with sterile dressing or clean pad (Fig. 12.6)

- Ensure the eyelashes are not folded in (inverted)
- Secure dressing with bandage
- Arrange transfer to hospital for further assessment
- **Trained personnel** may evert the eyelid to remove a foreign body

The ear

Lacerations

- Refer for specialized attention

Cauliflower ear

This is caused by bleeding, a result of a break in the cartilage. This results in swelling, scarring and permanent damage.

- Prompt treatment can reduce the deformity
- Apply a tight pressure bandage
- **Trained personnel** may drain blood with a sterile syringe

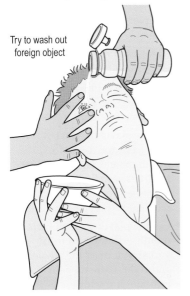

Try to wash out foreign object

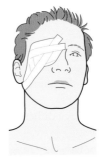

Fig. 12.5 Washing out the eye.

Fig. 12.6 Eye pad securely in place.

- Continue pressure following drainage

Perforated ear drum

- This may be caused by a violent blow to the ear
- The player complains of deafness and pain in the ear
- Refer for specialized assessment

MOUTH AND JAW

Red Zone

- **Swallowed tongue (see the ABC chapter)**
- **Broken tooth**
- **Broken jaw**
- **Severe laceration**

Amber Zone

- Serious mouth bleed
- Very swollen lip

Green zone

- **Minor mouth bleed**
- **Swollen lip**

What should I check for?

Speak to the player

- 'Are you OK?' 'Where did you get hit?'
- 'Where is the pain?' 'Did you hear a crack?'
- 'Do you have difficulty breathing?'
- 'Do you have any loose teeth?'
- Does the player have difficulty talking?

Problem identification

- A 'crack' usually indicates a fracture
- A lower face or jaw fracture may cause airway compromise and affect breathing
- A player with a broken jaw may not be able to talk

Observe

- Is there swelling/redness/ deformity/abrasion/ laceration?
- Compare with the other side – is there a difference?

Rule out serious injury

- Look for signs of facial fracture, severe head injury and spinal injury (see Chapter 17, page 164)

Touch (use gloves)

- Gently feel the facial bones for tenderness (?fracture)
- Examine jaw line for tenderness or a 'step' (there may be a fracture)
- Get the player to clench their teeth and assess for malalignment. Grip the upper teeth between finger and thumb and assess for tenderness or movement. Feel for loose teeth
- Get the player to open their mouth. Ask them to resist you as you push the jaw left and right. Extreme pain indicates a fracture
- Check the player's tongue for bleeding

Skills assessment

- Ask the player to blow out cheeks, smile and whistle (Fig. 12.1)

What should I do?

Talk to the player

- Reassure and explain what you are doing and why
- Minor injuries (Amber/green zone) may be dealt with on the pitch

Remove from the pitch

- **Do not** remove a player from the pitch unless it is safe to do so
- Removing the player allows you to reassess the situation and make a less pressured and more informed decision on the sideline
- When an injury is identified, assess whether it is safe to remove the player from the pitch without additional splinting or assistance

Emergency management

- ABC emergency management
- Emergency transfer to hospital if serious injury is suspected

Avoid further injury

- Get the player off the field of play for further assessment/management

Treat the problem

Mouth bleed

- Tilt head forward, allow blood to drain
- Avoid swallowing blood as this may cause vomiting
- Apply firm pressure to the area to stop bleeding
- Lacerations or cuts to the lips should be reviewed by a doctor

Broken jaw

- Gently apply a cold compress to reduce pain and limit swelling
- Manage as mouth bleed
- Refer to hospital

Broken/knocked-out tooth

- Gently push the tooth into the socket – make sure that you don't put the tooth in back to front
- Keep the tooth in place by pressing a gauze pad between the top and bottom teeth
- Get the player to hold the tooth firmly in place
- Send to hospital/dentist for further assessment/management
- If you cannot get the tooth into the socket, do not force it! Keep it moist in milk or saline

(or get the player to hold it under their tongue). It is important to get the player to a dentist or hospital as soon as possible

- If the player wears a gumshield, this may be used to hold the tooth in place

CUTS TO THE FACE

Lacerations in the so-called 'triangle of danger' (Fig. 12.7) always require specialized assessment.

Red Zone

- **Severe bleeding not stopping with pressure**
- **Cuts involving the eyeball**
- **Cuts where suspicion of underlying break in bone (fracture)**

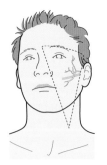

Fig. 12.7 The triangle of danger.

Amber Zone

- **Bleeding cuts**
- **Gaping cuts**
- **Cuts/abrasions contaminated with soil, grit or other foreign material**
- **Cuts in the danger zone of the face or crossing the border of the lip**
- **Cuts involving the eyelid**

Green zone

- **Superficial cuts, abrasions or friction burns**

What should I check for?

Speak to the player

- 'Are you OK?' 'How did it happen?'
- 'Where is the pain?' 'Did you hear a crack?'
- 'Do you feel numbness in your face?'
- 'Can you see me OK?'
- 'Are you up to date with your inoculations?'

Problem identification

- Numbness usually due to bruising or cut nerve
- If penetrating injury, what is the likely depth?

Observe

- Site, length and depth of cut
- Is it gaping?
- Is it actively bleeding?

- Is there dirt, grit or any other foreign body in the cut?
- Is there bruising, swelling?
- Is there asymmetry of the face?

Rule out serious injury

- Is there a head injury?
- Injury of the spine? (See Chapter 17, page 164)

Touch (use gloves)

- Feel for tenderness around the cut. Do you suspect a broken bone?

Skills assessment

- Ask the player to blow out their cheeks, smile, whistle, wrinkle forehead (Fig. 12.1)

What should I do?

Talk to the player

- Reassure and explain what you are doing and why

Remove from the pitch

- **Do not** remove a player from the pitch unless it is safe to do so
- Minor injuries (Green Zone) may be dealt with on the pitch
- Removing the player allows you to reassess the situation and make a less pressured and more informed decision on the sideline
- Assess whether it is safe to remove the player from the pitch without assistance

- All players with bleeding cuts must be removed from the field of play

Emergency management

- ABC of emergency management
- Stop bleeding with direct pressure
- Emergency transfer to hospital if serious injury is suspected

Avoid further injury

- Get the player off the field of play for further assessment/ management

Treat the problem

- Minor, superficial cuts and abrasions can be treated rapidly on the pitch or sideline. Clean with saline or tap water. Dry area with clean gauze and apply adhesive strips if required and/or Elastoplast. Vaseline can help prevent further bleeding
- If equipment and personnel are available, cuts can be cleaned and sutured by trained medical personnel
- Cover cuts with sterile dressing
- Keep the player sitting upright unless they are feeling faint

- Gaping cuts and deep cuts in the 'triangle of danger' (Fig. 12.7) and deep cuts of the lip and its border should be sent to hospital

- Remove gross debris by irrigating with saline or tap water
- Check that the player is up to date with their tetanus immunization.

Neck injuries

I Robertson, A R Poynton

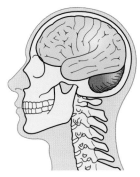

Fig. 13.1 The neck.

Neck injuries commonly occur in contact sports and should be treated with extreme caution.

Red Zone

- **Fracture**
- **Dislocation**
- **Disc disruption**

Amber Zone

- Muscle contusion/strain
- Stinger

Green zone

- **Minor blow to the neck**
- **Mild neck strain**

What should I check for?

Remember SPORTS and do not move the player immediately.

Speak to the player

- 'Can you hear me?' If the player is unconscious (**Red Zone Injury**), see the ABC chapter (p. 21)

- 'Where is the pain?'

- 'How sore is it?'

- 'Can you move all four limbs?'

- 'Can you feel all four limbs?'

Problem identification

Identify the extent of the injury by obtaining answers to the questions asked in the previous section. For example, the player may be complaining of neck pain and tingling or loss of sensation.

Observe

- Keep the player lying on the ground with their neck straight

- Make sure the player is breathing and observe for leg movement

- Look for any major abnormalities

Rule out serious injury

- Is the player unconscious or confused?

- Have they a weakness on one side of the body?

- Have they a severe headache?

If yes to any of these – serious head injury (**Red Zone Injury**).

- Can they move all four limbs?

- Have they full sensation?

If no to either of these – serious spinal injury (**Red Zone Injury**).

Touch for tenderness

- Ask the player to move all four limbs

- Touch the affected area lightly – Can they feel you touching them? Is the area very sore to touch?

- Can you feel any deformities in the affected area?

If the player has minimal pain and can move all four limbs ask them to move their head in all directions i.e. chin to each shoulder, chin to chest and look up to the sky (see Fig. 111.5, p. 80).

Skills assessment

- If player does not have full range of movement in the neck they should not play on

- If they have some stiffness they may be able to play on. Assess at half time and full time

Table 13.1 How serious is the neck injury

	Pain	Range of movement
Red Zone	+	↓
Amber Zone	–	↓
Amber Zone	+	–
Green Zone	–	–

What should I do?

Talk to the player
Explain to them what you are doing and reassure them.

Remove the player safely from the field of play
See Chapter 7.

Emergency transfer to hospital – if necessary
Follow spinal precautions instructions.

Avoid further injury
If in any doubt it is safest to place the player in a collar and remove them safely from the field of play.

Treatment

- Apply the collar as shown in Figures 7.1–7.5 (p. 47)
- If minor injury apply ice pack and advise player to rest
- Reassess at half-time and end of game

FRACTURES, DISLOCATIONS AND DISC DISRUPTIONS

What should I check for?

- Paralysis
- Loss of or altered sensation
- Severe pain

What should I do?

- ABC – see the ABC chapter (p. 21)
- Communicate with the player
- Do not move the player
- Apply collar and spinal board – trained personnel essential to protect neck and position player. See Chapter 7
- Compromised airway must be urgently managed – see the ABC chapter (p. 21)
- **Arrange for emergency transfer to hospital**

Red Zone

Amber Zone

MUSCLE CONTUSIONS/ STRAINS AND STINGERS

What should I check for?

- Can player feel and move all four limbs?
- How severe is the pain?
- Has the player got full range of movement – check by asking them to move their head in all directions, as described above

What should I do?

- Talk to and reassure the player
- Remove them safely from the field of play
- Apply collar if concerned
- Apply ice

If pain subsides and the player has full range of movement they can resume playing.

Stinger

This is like an electric shock that travels down the arm but fully resolves when the pressure is removed. It is usually a recurrent injury.

What should I check for?

- Pain in neck and shoulder travelling down into arm
- Does the arm or shoulder feel weak?

- Does the player feel pins and needles or numbness in the arm?
- Has the player got full range of movement?
- Does movement make the symptoms worse?

What should I do?

- Support the neck and remove the player safely from the pitch
- Get the player assessed by trained personnel

MINOR BLOW TO THE NECK AND MILD MUSCLE STRAIN

What should I check for?

- Has the player any neck pain?
- Has the player any loss of power/ sensation in the arms?
- Has the player full range of movement?

What should I do?

- Assess for range of movement and pain (see Fig. 11.5, p. 80)

If full range of movement and pain-free, the player can run it off and play on.

Upper limb injuries

M H Vioreanu, J H Mullett

INTRODUCTION

Upper limb injuries are very common in collision sports (e.g. rugby, ice-hockey) and in sports that use large ranges of motion of the arm (e.g. gymnastics, cricket). They occur mainly after falls on to an outstretched hand or a direct blow to the arm.

Injuries can range anywhere from a dislocation (shoulder, elbow) to a simple sprain or ligament damage.

We have divided the arm into three areas (Fig. 14.1):

- Shoulder area
- Elbow area
- Wrist and hand area

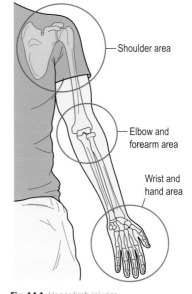

Fig. 14.1 Upper limb injuries.

Shoulder area

Elbow and forearm area

Wrist and hand area

INSTRUCTION

- Save life before limb
- Rule out neck injury

What should I check for?

Speak to the player

- Reassure the player
- Ask the player what happened. Get details of injury
- 'How did you land?'
- 'Did you feel/hear a crack?' (?Broken bone)
- 'Did you feel a snap or feel like you pulled a muscle?'
- 'Where is the pain?'
- 'Point to the sore area.'
- 'Does the pain go anywhere or is it in the same place?'
- 'Can you move your arm?'
- 'Do you have pins and needles?'

Problem identification

- A player in a lot of pain generally has a serious injury
- Most injuries of the arm are obvious enough
- A player will point to the area of soreness and complain of pulling a muscle or receiving a blow
- Asking how the injury happened will give clues as to what the injury is – for example, severe shoulder pain after direct impact

Observe

- Look at the arm in question and compare it to the other side
- Focus on where it is sore!
- Does the arm look different? Is it funny looking? (?Broken bone)
- Is the player holding their arm in a particular way?
- Is there any swelling of the arm? Look at the normal side
- Check for obvious bruising, grazes or bleeding

Rule out serious injury

Remember – pain in the arm can come from a neck injury.

- 'Can you move your arms?' (If not, this indicates a potential neck injury: see Ch. 13)
- Any pins and needles/ numbness in the arms? (If yes, treat as a neck injury)
- Can you see bone sticking out through the skin? (**Red Zone Injury**)
- Can you see blood spurting out from a wound? (**Red Zone Injury**)

Touch for tenderness

- Feel the area that was injured
- Is it swollen? Is it very sore to touch? (Does the player wince?)

- Is the arm red? Is it hot? This indicates inflammation

- Can you feel anything broken or unusual?

- Ask the player to move the joint

- Move the joint for the player. Is it very painful?

Skills assessment

- If the player is unable to fully move shoulder, elbow, wrist and fingers without pain (Amber Zone Injury), remove from field immediately and continue assessment on sideline

- Sometimes, the pain resolves rapidly and the player can perform sports-specific skills without discomfort

- Test joints above and below the injured area

- Do specific tests to assess each joint/muscle

- If the player can stand and demonstrate basic game skills, this is a good sign. This is a **Green Zone Injury** and the player may play on

What should I do?

Talk to the player

- Reassure the athlete, explain what is happening

Remove the player safely from the field of play

- If a neck injury is suspected, the player should have spine and back stabilization prior to transfer

- Any other injuries to the arm – ask the player to walk off the field with support

- If there are other injuries to the legs, etc., a stretcher is advised

Emergency transfer to hospital

- Any neck or spine injuries – ambulance

- Broken bones/dislocated – quickest possible means

Avoid further injury

- Immobilization of the injured arm

- Ensure no neck injury or other injury

- Any player who cannot perform basic skills runs the risk of doing more damage and should not continue (Amber Zone Injury)

Treatment

- Immobilization techniques (Figs 14.2–14.7)

- Application of ice

- Application of compressive bandage, if necessary

- Administration of painkillers (trained personnel only)

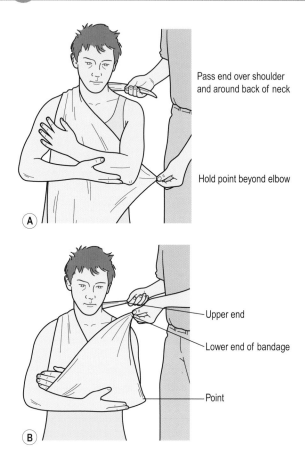

Pass end over shoulder and around back of neck

Hold point beyond elbow

Ⓐ

Upper end

Lower end of bandage

Point

Ⓑ

Fig. 14.2 Application of a broad arm sling.

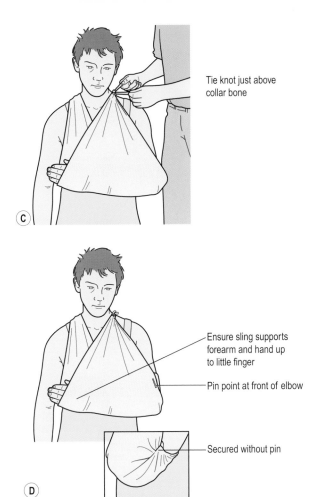

Tie knot just above collar bone

Ensure sling supports forearm and hand up to little finger

Pin point at front of elbow

Secured without pin

Fig. 14.2 *Continued.*

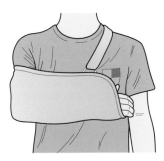

Fig. 14.3 Shoulder immobilizer.

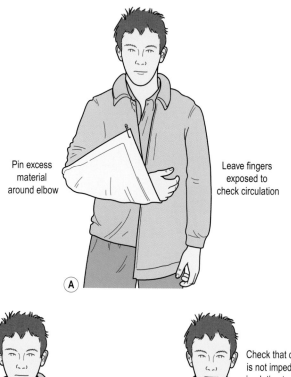

Pin excess
material
around elbow

Leave fingers
exposed to
check circulation

(A)

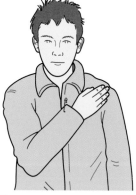

(B) Use a safety pin that is sturdy
enough to take weight of arm

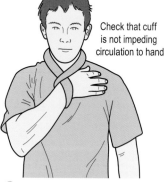

Check that cuff
is not impeding
circulation to hand

(C) Place hand in loop, where
it cannot slip out

Fig. 14.4 Improvised slings.

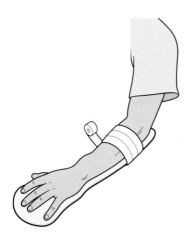

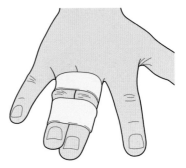

Fig. 14.7 Buddy strapping.

Fig. 14.5 Sam splint.

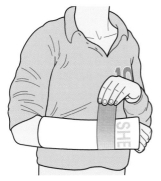

Fig. 14.6 Improvised splint. Place the injured arm inside a magazine and secure it with strapping.

SHOULDER AREA

Red Zone

- **Broken collar bone**
- **Dislocated shoulder**
- **Broken upper arm**

Amber Zone

- **Acromioclavicular joint injury**
- **Stinger**

Broken collar bone (Fig. 14.8)

What should I check for?

Speak to the player

- Reassure the player

Problem identification

- Ask the player to point to the sore area
- 'Where is the pain?'
- 'Did you hear a crack?'
- 'Can you move your shoulder?'

Observe

- Deformity of the collar bone
- Whether the player is anxious not to move the arm

Rule out serious injury

- Neck injury

Red Zone

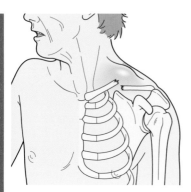

Fig. 14.8 Fractured clavicle.

Touch

- Extreme pain on light touch
- You may be able to feel the broken bone

Skills assessment

- The player is unable to move the shoulder

What should I do?

Talk to the player

- Reassure them

Remove safely from the field of play

- Support the injured arm
- Apply a broad arm sling

Emergency transfer to hospital

- **Send player to hospital** (by ambulance) in a seated position

Dislocated shoulder
(Fig. 14.9)

What should I check for?

Speak to the player

- Reassure the player
- 'Where is the pain?'
- 'Did you hear a crack?'
- 'Did you feel a pop?'

Problem identification

- How did it happen?
- The player will describe a feeling of the shoulder popping out
- The player will point to the pain

Observe

- Deformity of the injured shoulder
- Normally there is a fullness in the front of the shoulder
- You may notice a 'step' at the shoulder joint
- The player is anxious not to move the arm

Rule out serious injury

- Neck injuries

Touch for tenderness

- Extreme pain on light touch
- Feel for a 'step'. Follow the collar bone along to the edge. You will notice a step. Compare with the opposite side

Skills assessment

- The player is unable to move the shoulder

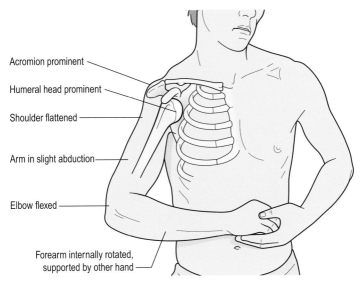

Acromion prominent

Humeral head prominent

Shoulder flattened

Arm in slight abduction

Elbow flexed

Forearm internally rotated,
supported by other hand

Fig. 14.9 Dislocated shoulder.

What should I do?

- Safely remove athlete from the pitch
- Do not attempt to relocate the shoulder on the pitch
- Support the arm
- Apply a broad arm sling
- **Send the player to hospital immediately**, in a seated position, with the shoulder supported

Broken upper arm (Fig. 14.10)

High energy is required to break the bone (e.g. motorbike racing, fall from a height, very high-impact tackle). In most cases the athlete knows the arm is broken, is in extreme pain and heard a 'snap'.

What should I check for?

Speak to the player

- Reassure the player
- 'Where is the pain?'
- 'Did you hear a snap or crack?'

Problem identification

- How did it happen?

Observe

- Deformity of the injured upper arm
- Look for any bleeding (torn skin)

Rule out serious injury

- Neck injury

Touch for tenderness

- Extreme pain on light touch
- The bone may 'tent' the skin

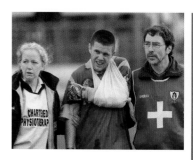

- Any weakness or numbness in the hand

Skills assessment

- The player will be unable to move the arm

What should I do?

- Remove the player safely from the field of play
- The injured arm should be supported in a splint
- Cover any visible bones or bleeding with a sterile gauze
- **Send the injured player to hospital immediately**

See Chapter 10 on broken bones.

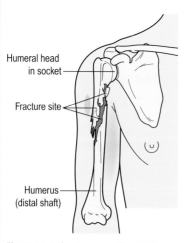

Humeral head
in socket

Fracture site

Humerus
(distal shaft)

Fig. 14.10 Broken upper arm (humerus).

Amber flags

- Pain out of proportion at simple examination
- Athlete not able to fully move their arm
- Decreased strength in the arm

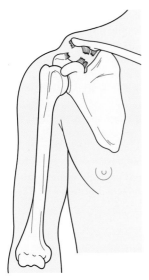

Fig. 14.11 Acromioclavicular joint disruption.

Acromioclavicular joint injury (Fig. 14.11)

The acromioclavicular joint is injured by falling on to the shoulder, elbow or an outstretched arm. It can range in severity, from a little bit of pain to complete rupture of the joint.

What should I check for?

Speak to the player

- Reassure the player
- 'Did you hear a snap or a pop?'

Problem identification

- How did it happen?

Observe

- Any swelling or lump around the shoulder
- Compare with the normal side

Rule out serious injury

Touch

- Pain at touch over the acromioclavicular joint
- Run your hand along the collar bone – a 'step' may be felt, which will be very tender. Compare with the normal side

Skills assessment

- Observe athlete performing basic sports skills

What should I do?

- **Remove athlete from competition**. Rest injured arm in broad arm sling
- Apply ice to the injured shoulder (Fig. 14.12)

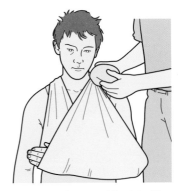

Fig. 14.12 Apply ice to an injured shoulder.

- Reassess patient and refer to sports medicine physician for further assessment and treatment
- See Figures 14.2–14.7 for immobilization techniques

Stinger

This injury is commonly encountered in contact sports (rugby, ice-hockey, Gaelic football), in which the shoulder takes the impact of a hit (Fig. 14.13), or in athletes with 'loose' shoulders. If we consider the shoulder joint as a ball and socket, it is the 'ball' that slips out of the 'socket' and goes back immediately. During this the nerves in the arm will tingle and give a 'dead arm' sensation. This is often referred to by players as 'electric shock' of the arm. (See also Neck Injuries, Ch. 80.)

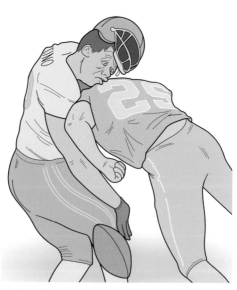

Fig. 14.13 American footballer receiving a 'stinger' in a tackle.

What should I check for?

Speak to the player

- Reassure the player
- 'Have you any pins and needles in your hand?'

Problem identification

- How did it happen?

Observe

- Shoulder looks normal, similar to the other side
- Limited movement in the shoulder

Rule out serious injury

- Do you have neck pain?

Touch

- Feel the shoulder – make sure it is not dislocated
- Ask the player to move their neck in all directions – is there any pain?
- Can the player put chin to chest, ear to shoulder, chin to shoulder?
- Touch the player's fingers to see if they can feel you

Skills assessment

- Observe the athlete performing basic sports skills

What should I do?

- Remove the player from competition
- Rest the injured arm in a broad arm sling
- Apply ice to the injured shoulder
- Occasionally, the symptoms may settle down and the player may play on
- Reassess patient and refer to sports medicine physician for further assessment and treatment

Guidelines on return to play

- The athlete must be pain free with full range of movement of the injured arm
- The athlete must be able to perform basic sport skills without pain
- No weakness in the injured arm

ELBOW AREA

Red Zone

- **Dislocated elbow**
- **Broken elbow/forearm**

Amber Zone

- **Painful elbow**
- **Badly bruised elbow/forearm**

Dislocated elbow (Fig. 14.14)

A dislocated elbow is not a common sports injury and is more likely to occur in high-impact sports. Deformity is obvious and the elbow is stiff. The player is in extreme pain and knows that the elbow is out of place.

Red Zone

What should I check for?

Speak to the player

- Reassure and ask questions
- The player will know that the elbow is out of place

Problem identification

- How did it happen?

Observe

- Obvious deformity of the elbow
- The player will be anxious not to move the arm

Rule out serious injury

- Neck injuries

Touch for tenderness

- Extreme pain with light touch and on attempts to move the elbow

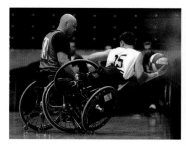

What should I do?

Talk to the player

Remove the player from the field immediately

Emergency transfer to hospital

Avoid further injury

- **Do not force the elbow in any position**

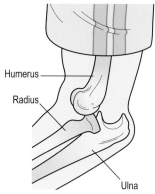

Fig. 14.14 Dislocated elbow.

Humerus

Radius

Ulna

- Keep the arm still

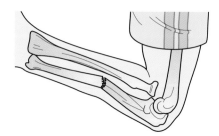

Fig. 14.15 Broken forearm.

- Keep the elbow in a comfortable position using a sling or towel

Broken elbow or forearm

(Fig. 14.15)

Most likely to occur in contact sports or motor sports as the result of a direct blow or fall on to the bent elbow. Deformity may be obvious in forearm fractures. It may be difficult to distinguish between a sprain and a fracture in the elbow.

What should I check for?

Speak to the player

- Reassure the player and ask questions
- 'Did you hear a crack?'
- In most cases the player knows the forearm is broken

Problem identification

- How did it happen?

Observe

- Obvious deformity of the forearm
- Player will be anxious not to move the elbow
- Look for any puncture wounds (open fracture)

Rule out serious injury

Touch

- Extreme pain with light touch or attempts to move the elbow

What should I do?

- Clean and dress wounds
- Immobilize elbow/forearm in comfortable position
- Apply a splint – keep arm elevated in a sling (see Figs 14.2–14.6)
- **Send to hospital**

Amber flags

- Pain out of proportion at simple examination
- Athlete not able to fully move their arm
- Decreased strength in the arm

Painful elbow

Over-straightening of the elbow occurs when the elbow is bent back the wrong way. This type of injury will occur more frequently in contact sports such as rugby or certain martial arts, e.g. jujitsu. The pain is caused when the elbow is forced to bend the wrong way, causing damage to the ligaments and structures of the elbow.

Amber Zone

What should I check for?

Speak to the player

- 'Where is the pain?'
- 'How painful is your elbow?'
- 'Does it feel out of place?'

Problem identification

- How did it happen?

Observe

- No obvious deformity
- Pain with movement of the elbow

Rule out serious injury

Touch for tenderness

- The elbow will be sore to touch

Skills assessment

- The player will not be able to complete basic sports skills

What should I do?

- Remove the player from competition. Rest the injured elbow in a broad arm sling (see Fig. 14.2)
- Apply ice to the injured elbow
- Strapping should be applied, preferably by trained personnel, to prevent further bending of the elbow
- Reassess the player and refer for specialist review, further assessment and treatment

Badly bruised elbow/forearm

Bruising around the upper arm and forearm is relatively common in contact sports after a direct blow. A large, painful, swollen bruise that develops within 30 minutes may indicate a more serious injury.

What should I check for?

Speak to the player

- 'Where is the pain?'
- 'How painful is your elbow?'
- 'Can you move the fingers? Is that painful?'

Problem identification

- How did it happen?

Observe

- Observe bruise; red to bluish colour
- Observe swelling

Rule out serious injury

- Rule out more serious injuries, such as elbow dislocation, forearm fracture

Touch for tenderness

- Painful to touch

Skills assessment

- The player will not be able to complete basic sports skills

What should I do?

- Remove the player from competition. Rest the bruised forearm in a broad arm sling

- Apply ice to the injured forearm
- Reassess the player and refer to specialist for further assessment and treatment

Guidelines on return to play

- The athlete must be pain free with full range of movement of the injured arm
- The athlete must be able to perform basic sport skills without pain
- No weakness in the injured arm

WRIST AND HAND AREA

Red Zone

- **Broken wrist**

Amber Zone

- **Dislocated finger**
- **Mallet ('jammed') finger**

Broken wrist (Fig. 14.16)

Wrist fracture is a commonly encountered injury in contact sports. It is frequently caused by a fall on to an outstretched arm or a direct blow to the wrist.

What should I check for?

Speak to the player

- 'Where is the pain?'
- 'How painful is the wrist?'
- 'Can you move the fingers? Is that painful?'
- 'Do you feel any pins and needles in your fingers?'

Problem identification

- How did it happen?

Observe

- Obvious deformity ('dinner fork') in some cases
- Observe swelling

Rule out serious injury

Touch for tenderness

- Painful when touching/ palpating the wrist

Skills assessment

- Pain with movement of the wrist
- Athlete not able to complete basic sports skills

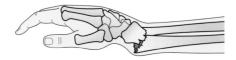

Fig. 14.16 Broken wrist.

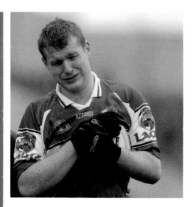

What should I do?

- Remove the player from competition. Rest the bruised wrist in a broad arm sling
- Apply ice to the injured wrist
- **Send the player to hospital** (ambulance) in sitting position with shoulder supported in a sling
- See Figures 14.2–14.6 for immobilization techniques

Dislocated finger

(Fig. 14.17)

This injury is encountered in many sporting events. It is very painful. It is often relatively easy for a rescuer with the right training to put such a digit back into place ('reduce' it), bringing quick relief to the injured person

What should I check for?

Speak to the player
- Reassure the player
- Explain what you want to do (relocate the finger – see below)

Problem identification
- How did it happen?

Observe
- Obvious deformity

Rule out serious injury

Touch for tenderness

Skills assessment

What should I do?

- Remove the player from competition
- Immobilize the painful finger (see Fig. 14.7)
- **Send the player to hospital**

Relocating the finger back in place (for qualified personnel)

1. Explain each step to the player and reassure them
2. Hold the finger firmly with both hands, keeping it in a

Amber Zone

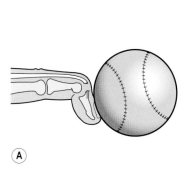 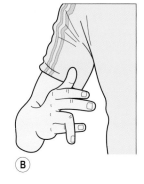

Fig. 14.17 Dislocated finger.

slightly bent position. Do this by placing one hand below the base of the dislocated joint and the other at the end of the tip of the finger

3. Pull gently on the tip of the finger along the line in which the bones normally lie, as if trying to lengthen it in a straight line, while simultaneously pushing the joint back into place with your other hand

4. Splint the finger by taping it to the neighbouring digit, cushioning the splint with a gauze pad between the two fingers. Do not put tape directly on the joint

5. **Send the player to hospital** for an X-ray and further treatment and follow-up.

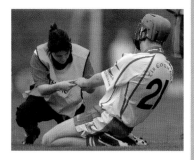

Mallet finger (Fig. 14.18)

This injury is very common in ball sports. It is caused by the direct impact of a ball on the top of a finger or snagging of a finger in a jersey.

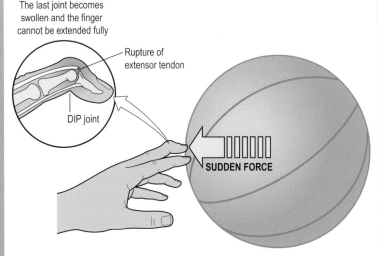

The last joint becomes swollen and the finger cannot be extended fully

Rupture of extensor tendon

DIP joint

SUDDEN FORCE

Fig. 14.18 Mallet finger.

What do I check for?

Speak to the player

- 'What happened?'
- 'Where did the ball land?'
- 'Did you hear or feel a snap?'

Problem identification

- This should be obvious!

Observe

- Look at the finger side-on. Compare it with the same finger on the opposite hand. The injured digit will sag beyond the joint. The player will be unable to straighten the last joint in the finger

Rule out serious injury

Touch (use gloves)

- Feel the joint – it will be tender and swollen
- Feel the rest of the joints in the finger for any tenderness

Skills assessment

What should I do?

- Remove the player from competition
- Immobilize the painful finger using a splint to keep the finger straight (Fig. 14.19) – a lollipop stick is very handy!
- **Send the player to hospital for an X-ray and further follow-up**

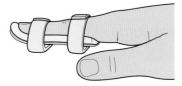

Fig. 14.19 Splinted mallet finger.

Guidelines on return to play

Most finger injuries do not require substitution. The player may complain of swollen joint which can be quite painful. The most important thing to do is observe the finger compared to the others:

• Does the finger look right?
• Is it straight?
• Can the player move the finger?

If yes, the player can play on. It is often advisable to strap the two fingers together (Figure 14.7), as this makes it easier to continue to play. Assess the player after the game.

M H Vioreanu, S P Gaine

INTRODUCTION

Three main scenarios may arise:

- 'I can't breathe – I was not hit!' (Fig. 15.1)

- 'I have pain in my chest – I was not hit!' (Fig. 15.2)

- 'I can't breathe and I have chest pain – I was hit!' (Fig. 15.3)

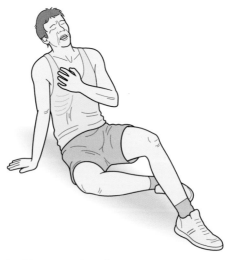

Fig. 15.1 Sudden breathlessness – no trauma!

Fig. 15.2 Pain in chest – no trauma!

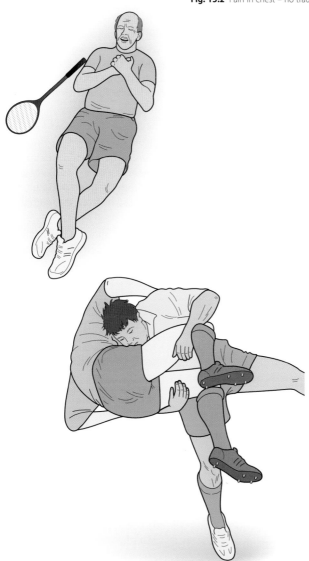

Fig. 15.3 I can't breathe and I have pain in my chest – I was hit.

APPROACHING THE PLAYER WITH BREATHING/CHEST PROBLEMS

What should I check for?

Speak to the player

- 'Can you tell me what happened?'
  - 'Were you hit?'
- 'Do you have any pain?'
  - 'Where is the pain?'
  - 'Does the pain go anywhere else?'
  - 'Is it worse on breathing?'
  - 'Do you feel short of breath?'
- 'Has this ever happened before?'
- 'Do you have any breathing problems?'
  - 'Are you asthmatic?'
- 'Do you have any heart problems?'
- 'Are you taking any medications?'

Problem identification

- The mechanism of injury will give a good clue as to the cause of the problem
- By speaking with the player you can get a good indication of how serious the problem is

If a player can't speak or is extremely out of breath it is a serious condition (**Red Zone Injury**)– go to the ABC chapter (p. 21).

- Contact – 'I was hit' – more than likely a muscular or bony injury
- No contact – 'I was not hit' – WARNING – There may be a breathing condition or heart condition. Take extreme caution!
- The site of the pain will give a clue as to the cause
  - Central Chest Pain – Behind the breast bone – Is likely to be from the heart or lungs, but can also be from the stomach or be caused by anxiety
  - Pain to either side to rib cage – Most likely to be from the lung
- Type of pain
  - Crushing pain – constant, unrelenting – likely to be from the heart
  - Pain on breathing likely to be from the lung or ribs
- Does the pain go anywhere?
  - A pain running down the left arm or into the jaw – **always think Heart Attack!**
  - Tightness across the chest going into the back may be from the lungs or heart – **Caution!**
- Other illnesses or medications
  - It is very important to know if a player has a known condition
  - Find out about any medication – the player may

INFORMATION

Signs and symptoms of 'breathing problems'

- Rapid deep breathing
- Noisy breathing
- Flaring nostrils
- Dizziness or faintness
- Anxiety or confusion
- Straining muscles: neck, face, chest, abdomen
- Blue discoloration – lips, face
- Numbness or tingling – hands/ feet
- Spasm of fingers and toes

If player has one of the above problems treat them as an emergency – see the ABC chapter (p. ••).

have it with them and it may be very useful to treat them

Observe

- Look at the player's general appearance, position, ability to breathe and speak

Rule out serious injury

Airway problem or respiratory arrest (Red Zone Injury):

- If player is able to speak normally, the airway is probably OK
- Establish if the player is able to breathe on their own
- Make sure to check the airway if they are unable to speak – **go immediately to** the ABC chapter (p. 21)

Touch for tenderness

- Feel for point tenderness of the chest
- Place your hand on either side of the chest wall to confirm they are moving equally with each breath
- Feel over the airway to make sure it is in the centre of the neck
- If an injury is located, feel the ribs to check any breaks or abnormality – if found, this is a **Red Zone Injury**

Skills assessment

- Assess the player's ability to breathe while exercising, preferably on the side of the pitch
- If the player continues to struggle to breathe, and is not just winded or 'out of puff', they must come off to be assessed further

If a breathing problem is identified, remove player from the play immediately.

What should I do?

A player with a serious breathing problem or chest injury needs to be removed immediately from the field of play for assessment and treatment. These are **Red Zone Injuries** until proven otherwise!

Talk to the player

- Reassure the player, explain what is happening

- Act calmly and with assurance
- By talking to the player, establish their capacity to breathe

Remove the player safely from the field of play

- The player should walk off the pitch with assistance
- If the player is seriously injured they should be taken off on a stretcher

Emergency transfer to hospital

- Any serious chest injury should be transferred to hospital by ambulance if available or as soon as possible by other means

Avoid further injury

- Remove the player from any environment that could worsen the breathing problem, e.g. smoke, cold air, fog
- Perform ongoing assessment of the player's state
- **DO NOT leave the player alone**

Treatment

- Keep player at rest in a comfortable environment
- Place player in a sitting position. It helps if the player can support themselves on their forearms when sitting – this eases their efforts to expand the chest
- Continue to talk with the player

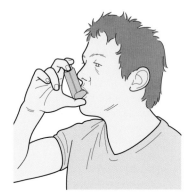

Fig. 15.4 Use of a beta-agonist inhaler.

- If a player stops speaking or is unable to speak, check that the airway is open
- If in doubt at any stage, go to the ABC chapter (p. 21)
- Administer oxygen if available
- Assist player with medication (beta-agonist inhaler – salbutamol, etc.) if they are familiar with it (Fig. 15.4)
- Cover the player to conserve body heat
- Continue to monitor the player and provide emotional support

 INFORMATION

Adequate breathing = 'breathing that is sufficient to support life'

- Easy and effortless
- Able to speak full sentences
- Normal respiration rate (12–20 breaths/minute)

'I CAN'T BREATHE – I WAS NOT HIT'

Red Zone

- **Severe asthma attack**
- **Anaphylaxis**
- **Collapsed lung (Spontaneous pneumothorax) (Fig. 15.1)**
- **Epiglottitis**

Amber Zone

- Mild or moderate asthma attack
- Chest infection/bad cough
- Hyperventilation

Green zone

- **Athlete out of shape**

Severe asthma attack

Exercise induced asthma is very common. The asthma attack usually occurs in the first 5–10 minutes after starting exercising or 5–10 minutes following exercise, and may last up to 30 minutes. Fast, hard breathing, coughing, wheezing and a tight chest are signs of an asthma attack, which can be very serious, even life-threatening. As many as 10–20% of all athletes will experience some form of asthma attack when exercising in cold, dry air (e.g. cross-country skiing, ice-hockey).

What should I check for?

Speak to the player

- What happened?
- Did you get hit?
- Are you having trouble breathing?
- Do you have asthma?
  - Where's your inhaler?
- Do you have any pain?
- Does it hurt to take a deep breath in?

Problem identification
By talking to the player, decide upon the severity of the attack

- A player severely out of breath, unable to speak, extremely agitated or panicking is likely to be having a serious attack. They need to calm down, take their medication and be sent to hospital

Observe

- Observe the way the player is breathing
  - The player is anxious and in obvious respiratory distress
  - The player is breathing rapidly (fast rate) – easy inhalation and forced, noisy expiration (wheezing)
  - The player is using other muscles to breathe –

abdominal breathing, straining of neck muscles, and sucking in of cheeks

- The player may have a bluish tint to their skin, especially around the lips

Rule out serious injury

- Make sure the airway is open
- Ensure that the player is able to speak

If the airway closes or the player can no longer breathe, go immediately to the ABC chapter (p. 21).

Skills assessment

If the player is suffering from a chest injury, it is advisable to remove them from competition. Only players with minor injuries should be allowed to return to action.

What should I do?

Talk to the player

Breathing difficulties and chest pain cause extreme anxiety and distress.

- Act calmly and with assurance – tension and anxiety makes an asthma attack worse
- Try to focus the player on calm, controlled breathing

Remove the player safely from the field of play

Avoid further injury

- Stopping activity will reduce the stress on the heart and lungs
- Remove the player from an environment that may cause breathing difficulties – cold, dry, foggy air

Emergency transfer

Call for an ambulance if necessary.

Treatment

- Give oxygen
- Place the player in a seated position
- Attempt to give an inhaler – salbutamol or equivalent (Fig. 15.4)
- Send patient to the hospital by ambulance, or get the player to hospital by the quickest means possible if an ambulance is not available
- Encourage slow deep breaths

Do not leave the player unattended!

Anaphylaxis/anaphylactic shock (see also Ch. 6)

Anaphylaxis is an extreme allergic reaction that can be life-threatening. Anaphylaxis may be associated with widespread itching and the same signs and symptoms as asthma. Although not commonly encountered, athletes may have an anaphylactic reaction to a substance – an allergen – which could be anything from eating certain nuts through being bitten or stung by an insect to receiving antibiotic medication.

What should I check for?

Speak to the player

- Make sure the player can speak! A player who cannot speak indicates a swollen airway. This is a **Red Zone Injury** – go immediately to the ABC chapter (p. 21)
- 'What happened?'
- 'Are you having trouble breathing?'
- 'Did you get stung by anything?'
- 'Did you eat anything strange?'
- 'Do you have any known allergies?'
- 'Do you have any itching sensation?'
- 'Has this ever happened before?'
- 'Do you take any medications?'

Problem identification

- Anaphylactic reactions are not always very obvious
- A player will often complain of feeling very hot and bothered

- They may complain of swelling and feeling congested
- They are often agitated and irritable

Observe

- The player may be anxious – this could be respiratory distress
- Their breathing may be noisy or 'whistling'
- If they complain of an itch or soreness on their skin – check for an insect bite or rash
- Sometimes the rash is on the player's chest or back and is not very obvious. Remove the player from the field of play and check these areas if they complain of itchiness there
- Look out for raised areas of skin, redness, blotchiness, blistering or swelling

Rule out serious injury.

- Make sure airway is open

Touch for tenderness

- Feel the player's forehead to see if they have a temperature
- Touch any area of skin that feels itchy
  - Feel for swelling
  - Feel for any raised areas on the skin which may indicate a rash
- Feel under the angle of the jaw for any swelling of the glands

- If a bite is identified you may feel the 'stinger' – be careful not to get stung yourself!

Skills assessment
The player is not able to continue physical activity.

What should I do?

Talk to the player
Act calmly and with assurance. Tension and anxiety makes breathing worse.

Remove the player safely from the field of play

Emergency transfer
Call for an ambulance.

Avoid further injury

- Stopping activity will reduce the stress on the heart and lungs

- Remove the player from an environment that may cause breathing difficulties – cold, dry, foggy air

- Remove the allergen (the stinger of an insect bite) – take care not to harm yourself!

Treatment
According to the severity of an anaphylaxis attack, treat as follows:

- If the player has difficulties breathing, generalized rash and swollen lips

- Call for an ambulance
- Give the player oxygen if available
- Use injectable adrenaline if available (see Fig. 6.3, p. 43)
- Reassess frequently – if the player stops speaking or the airway closes go immediately to the ABC chapter (p. 21)

- A player with anaphylaxis but no breathing difficulties
  - Place athlete in sitting position
  - Give antihistamine medication if available
  - Observe every 15 minutes

 INFORMATION

Insect bites and stings

- The swelling associated with an insect bite may be dramatic and frightening
- Because the sting of a bee remains in the skin, it can continue to inject venom for up to 20 minutes after the bee has gone
- You should gently attempt to remove sting attached to the skin/muscle by scraping the skin with the edge of a sharp, stiff object such as a credit card.
- **Do not leave the player unattended.**

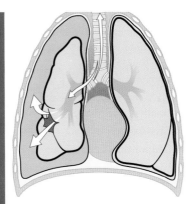

Fig. 15.5 Collapsed lung (spontaneous pneumothorax).

Collapsed lung (Spontaneous pneumothorax)

Spontaneous pneumothorax is a collection of air between the outside surface of the lung and the inside surface of the chest wall causing the lung to collapse (Fig. 15.5). Spontaneous means there is no injury to the chest or lung. It usually occurs in tall, thin men between the ages of 20 and 40. Competition at high altitude may be a contributory factor. **Symptoms often begin suddenly and can occur while exercising or resting. This is a potentially life-threatening condition for the athlete and needs to be dealt with urgently by a doctor.**

What should I check for?

Speak to the player
- 'What happened?'
- 'Are you having trouble breathing?'
- 'Did you get hit?'
- 'Do you have any pain in the chest?'
- 'Where is the pain?'
- 'Does it hurt to breathe in?'
- 'Has this ever happened before'

Problem identification
- The player will complain of a sharp pain and localize it to one side of the chest
- The pain is worse on taking a deep breath
- Tall males are more likely to develop spontaneous pneumothorax
- This problem can be recurrent, so it is important to determine whether it has happened before. If it has, the player will know all about it!

Observe
Observe the way the athlete is breathing:
- May be anxious and in respiratory distress
- Watch the movement of the rib cage – one side will not move compared to the other
- Watch to see if the player is using other muscles to breathe

– straining of neck muscles, sucking in of the cheeks and tummy as they try to get more air in!

• Look for a bluish tint to the skin, especially around the lips – this indicates low oxygen levels in the blood

Rule out serious injury.

• Make sure airway is open

Touch for tenderness

• Feel player's 'wind pipe'. In severe cases this is not in the middle

• Feel both sides of the player's chest to see if they are moving equally with each breath. No movement on one side would suggest a collapsed lung on that side

Skills assessment

• The player is not able to continue physical activity

What should I do?

Talk to the player
Act calmly and with assurance – Tension and anxiety makes breathing worse

Remove the player safely from the field of play

Emergency transfer
Call for an ambulance

Avoid further injury

• Stopping activity will reduce the stress on the heart and lungs

• Remove the player from an environment which may cause breathing difficulties – cold, dry, foggy air

Treatment

• Place the player in a seated position

• Give oxygen

• Call for medical assistance

• Large collections of air crushing the lungs need insertion of a chest drain so **urgently send patient to hospital**

• A doctor may try to decompress the lung by inserting a needle into the chest. This should not be attempted by anyone without prior experience!

Epiglottitis

Epiglottitis is a disorder caused by inflammation of the cartilage that covers the windpipe. It is most common in children. Although rare, epiglottitis can occur in normal adults. Because it is rare in adults, it may be easily overlooked. The epiglottis (the flap of cartilage at the back of the tongue that closes off the windpipe when swallowing) swells and can obstruct breathing. Respiratory distress increases rapidly as the epiglottis swells. This is a life-threatening disease that begins with fever and sore throat.

What should I check for?

Speak to the player

- 'What happened?'
- 'Are you having trouble breathing?'
- 'Do you have a sore throat?'
- 'Do you feel very unwell?'
- 'Do you feel hot and sweaty?'
- 'Has this ever happened before?'

Problem identification

- This problem is more often seen in children
- The players will often have a fever and sore throat
- The player may complain of feeling as if they have a temperature – hot and bothered – more than just hot and sweaty with exercise

Observe

Observe the way the player is breathing:

- The player will be anxious, in respiratory distress and becoming progressively more short of breath
- The player may be using other muscles to breathe (neck, face) – nasal flaring
- Player may have a bluish tinge to the skin, especially around the lips

Rule out serious injury

- Make sure the airway is open and that nothing is obstructing it
- If at any stage the player is unable to talk or is having increasing difficulty breathing, go immediately to the ABC chapter (p. 21)

Skills assessment

The player is not able to continue with physical activity.

What should I do?

Talk to the player

Act calmly and with assurance – tension and anxiety make breathing more difficult.

Remove the player safely from the field of play

Emergency transfer

Call for an ambulance

Avoid further injury

- Stopping activity will reduce the stress on the heart and lungs
- Remove the player from an environment which may cause breathing difficulties – cold, dry, foggy air

Treatment

- Call for medical assistance
- Sit the player upright
- Encourage deep slow breaths
- Give the player oxygen

• Do **not** attempt to clear the airway by sticking anything into the mouth. This could make the problem worse by causing the airway to swell further

• **Urgently send player by ambulance to hospital**

• **Do not leave the player unattended!**

Mild or moderate asthma attack

Asthma attacks are common during sport. Thankfully, most attacks are mild or moderate and the player can return to play following some minor treatment.

What should I check for?

Speak to the player

• 'What happened?'

• 'Did you get hit?'

• 'Are you having trouble breathing?'

• 'Do you have asthma?'
  • 'Where's your inhaler?'

• 'Do you have any pain?'

• 'Does it hurt to take a deep breath in?'

Problem identification
By talking to player decide upon severity of the attack

• A player severely out of breath, unable to speak, extremely agitated or panicking is likely to be having a serious attack. They need to calm down, take their medication and be sent to hospital

• A player suffering a mild attack should be able to speak full sentences but will complain of some tightness across their chest

• Players with asthma are usually very familiar with the feeling of an attack and will frequently search for their inhaler for relief

Observe
Observe the way the player is breathing:

• The player is slightly caught for breath and somewhat agitated

• Their breathing is somewhat strained with an increased breathing rate

Rule out serious injury

• Make sure the airway is open

• Ensure the player is able to speak and keep a close observation to recognize any worsening of the condition

Touch for tenderness

• Feel the movement of the chest wall

- Make sure both sides are moving equally

Skills assessment

The player should be able to return to activity once their breathing improves.

What should I do?

Talk to the player

- Act calmly and with assurance – Tension and anxiety makes asthma attack worse

Remove the player safely from the field of play – if necessary

Emergency transfer

Only necessary if the player's condition worsens

Avoid further injury

- Stopping activity will reduce the stress on the heart and lungs
- Remove the player from an environment which may cause breathing difficulties – cold, dry, foggy air

Treatment

According to severity of attack (based on ability to speak), treat as follows:

- Player with obvious wheezing/difficulties speaking full sentences
  - Temporarily remove the player to the side line
  - Place them in a seated position

- Give them their inhaler (Fig. 15.4)
- Observe for a few minutes to see if they improve
- Exercise the player on the sideline. If there is no change, the player can return to play with close observation

Chest infection/bad cough

An infection affects the player's lungs, either the larger airways or the smaller air sacs. Secretions build up in the chest and make it more difficult for the player to breathe. As a player starts to exercise they become short of breath more easily as they cannot get as much oxygen in.

This condition could present before or during the competition.

What should I check for?

Speak to the player

- 'What happened?'
- 'Did you get hit?'
- 'Are you having trouble breathing?'
- 'Do you have a cough?'
- 'Do you have asthma?'
- 'Do you have any pain?'
- 'Do you feel hot or cold?'

Problem identification

- A player will normally indicate that they have a cough

- They will feel caught on breathing
- The player may also complain of feeling unwell, with fevers or chills

Observe

- Observe the way the player is breathing
- Listen to their breathing – it may sound 'wheezy' or you may hear a 'rattle'
- The player may be coughing or bringing up phlegm

Rule out serious injury

- Make sure the player's airway is open
- Rule out an asthma attack
- Rule out an anaphylactic reaction

Touch for Tenderness

Feel the player's forehead for a temperature.

Skills assessment

The player should not play on with a chest infection.

What should I do?

Talk to the player

Act calmly and with assurance – tell the player they are coming off.

Remove the player safely from the field of play – if necessary

Emergency transfer

Only necessary if the player's condition worsens

Avoid further injury

- Stopping activity will reduce the stress on the heart and lungs
- Remove the player from an environment which may cause breathing difficulties – cold, dry, foggy air

Treatment

- Bring the player off the field of play
- Keep them warm
- If the player is coughing:
  - Sit them forward
  - Gently tap them on the back to encourage them to bring the phlegm up
  - Tell them to spit the phlegm out
- Give the player plenty of fluids to drink
- Refer them to a medical professional for further investigations and treatment

Hyperventilation

Hyperventilation is fast, shallow breathing. Anxiety and stress are the most common causes. It is commonly seen in players suffering from overtraining syndrome or prior to an important competition.

- This condition can occur before or during the competition

Speak to the player

- 'What happened?'
- 'Were you hit?'
- 'Are you having trouble breathing?'
- 'Do you have asthma?'
- 'Do you have any pain?'
- 'Do you have any medical problems?'
  - Are you taking any medications?'
- 'Do you have any tingling in your hands?'

Problem identification

- Players will be slow to admit to being anxious or nervous
- The important thing to do is to make sure they have no other conditions and no pain
- The player may look frightened or panicked as they struggle to control their breathing
- Tingling in the hands is a side effect of hyperventilation

Observe

- Observe the way the player is breathing
  - The player's breathing is fast and shallow
  - The player may be anxious and distressed as this is a frightening experience

- Make sure the player doesn't have a bluish tinge to their lips
- Sometimes the player will experience a 'panic attack'
- Make sure their chest is moving with each breath

Rule out serious injury

- Make sure the airway is open
- Rule out an asthma attack
- Rule out an anaphylaxis reaction

Touch for tenderness

- Feel the player's forehead for a temperature
- Feel the player's chest to make sure both sides are moving equally with each breath

Skills assessment

- The player will not be able to continue physical activity when having an attack and should be removed to the sideline
- Quick recovery occurs in many cases and the player can resume play when their breathing settles down

What should I do?

Talk to the player

- Act calmly and with assurance – it is important to take charge of this situation. Tell the player to relax and calm their breathing down

- Anxiety will only make the breathing worse
- Try to get the player to breathe with you – count your breaths

Remove the player safely from the field of play – if necessary

- By taking the player off the field of play you can remove them temporarily from their source of anxiety
- Take them to somewhere quiet

Emergency transfer
Only necessary if the player's condition worsens.

Avoid further injury

- Stopping activity will reduce the stress on the heart and lungs
- Remove the player from an environment which may cause breathing difficulties – cold, dry, foggy air

Treatment

- Get the player to sit down on a chair and remove anyone else from the treatment area. The more people, the more potential for anxiety
- Talk with the player, tell them what is happening:
  - 'You need to slow your breathing. The more tense you are, the faster you'll breathe'
  - 'Try to relax! This will soon pass. Nothing bad is going to happen'
- Keep the player warm
- If the player's breathing is not settling – get the player to breathe into a paper bag, or whatever bag is available. The theory is that rebreathing into a paper bag will allow the person to replace the carbon dioxide 'blown off' while hyperventilating
- If the player's condition is not improving despite treatment, contact trained medical personnel

Player out of shape

This is by far the most common reason for players complaining that they can't breathe. It is normally very obvious that they are unfit, and they will tell you this, although sometimes reluctantly!

Make sure there are no underlying problems such as asthma by going through the SPORTS questionnaire at the start of the chapter.

The only treatment is to get **fit**!

'I HAVE PAIN IN MY CHEST – I WAS NOT HIT'

Red Zone

- Cardiac chest pain
- Non-cardiac chest pain

Any chest pain represents a potentially serious condition. Although chest pain may be cardiac or non-cardiac, it is often difficult to distinguish between the two. A person with pain in their chest without contact should be treated as having a cardiac event until proven otherwise. Medical professionals should be contacted immediately to deal with this scenario.

Cardiac chest pain

Chest pain originating from the heart is not common among athletes. Chest pain without trauma is a medical emergency. A player over the age of 35 having chest pain without an injury to the chest is more likely to be experiencing a 'heart attack'. This is a general term indicating a failure of the blood supply to the heart muscle that damages or destroys a portion of the heart.

Whenever you suspect a player is having a heart attack, seek help from a medical professional or transfer the player urgently to hospital.

What should I check for?

Speak to the player

- 'What happened?'
- 'Did you get hit?'
- 'Do you have pain in your chest?'
- 'Does the pain go anywhere?' (e.g. jaws, neck, left arm)
- 'Does your heart beat feel unusual?'
- 'Do you have any heart problems?'
- 'Has this ever happened before?'
- 'Are you taking any medication?'
  - 'Do you have a spray for under your tongue?'
- 'Do you have trouble breathing?'
- 'Do you feel hot and sweaty?'
- 'Do you feel sick?'

Problem identification

- The player looks very unwell and is in some distress
- Consider the player's age – a heart attack is more likely to happen in older players over the age of 35
- They will complain of feeling hot and sweaty, more so than the normal for playing sport!
- Pain going down the left arm, into the jaw or into the back is a classic sign of cardiac pain

- It is important to determine if the player has a known history of heart problems or is on medication, particularly a GTN (glyceryl trinitrate) spray

- Difficulty breathing, nausea and light-headedness can be associated with cardiac chest pain

- A player may complain of an irregular heart beat – palpitations – a feeling that their heart is going to beat out of their chest! This may represent an arrhythmia, which may be life-threatening

Observe

INFORMATION

Signs and symptoms of heart attack

- Early symptoms: upper abdominal sensation of pressure and burning. At this stage symptoms are often mistaken for indigestion

- As the attack worsens, the pain may localize behind the breast bone and move to either the arm or the shoulder (usually the left one). Pain may extend to the hand, neck, jaw, teeth, upper back or upper abdomen

- Chest pain may be accompanied by other symptoms that suggest a heart attack: shortness of breath, nausea, sweating and weakness

- The pain may diminish when physical exertion ends or when the player takes a spray under their tongue.

When a player is experiencing some of the symptoms described in the box, be highly suspicious of a heart attack.

What will I see?

- Clutching chest or rubbing chest

- Sweaty, pale, clammy – the player may have a 'greyish' appearance

- Short of breath – unable to complete sentences

Rule out serious injury

This is a very serious injury!

- Make sure the player's airway is open

- At any stage if the player becomes unresponsive go immediately to the ABC chapter (p. 21)

Touch for tenderness

- Touch the player's forehead to see if they have a temperature. The skin will feel clammy

- Feel for the player's pulse (see page 29)

- The pulse may be very fast or thready – difficult to feel with a low volume

- The pulse may feel very irregular – arrhythmias – irregular heart beat

Skills assessment

This is not appropriate in this situation. The player will not be able to continue physical activity.

What should I do?

Talk to the player
Act calmly and with assurance – tell the player they are coming off.

Remove the player safely from the field of play
If the incident happens on the field of play, the player should be removed to the sidelines for further treatment. The player can be removed by stretcher or walking with assistance depending on the severity of their symptoms.

Emergency transfer

- **The player should be taken to hospital immediately**, ideally by ambulance but, if this is not available, by any other means

- When calling an ambulance specify that you think the player is having a heart attack – they will send a cardiac ambulance!

Avoid further injury

- Stopping activity will reduce the stress on the heart and lungs

- Remove the player from an environment that may cause breathing difficulties – cold, dry, foggy air

Treatment

- Call for help

- Seek medical assistance

- Keep the player sitting up at 45°

- Give oxygen if available

- Give the player aspirin (300 mg), if available, and tell them to chew it

- If the player has a spray, you can give them a spray under their tongue. Tell the player to lift their tongue. Spray two good sprays under the tongue. Repeat as necessary

  - GTN spray may give rise to a severe headache!

  - Some patients may have oral tablets instead of the spray

- Monitor the player at all times; keep talking to them to ensure they are conscious

- Always assess the airway to make sure it remains open – if in doubt go immediately to the ABC chapter (p. ●●)

- A doctor on the scene may give some pain relief to help with the chest pain

- Get the player to the hospital as soon as possible. All the above measures can be carried out in transit

INFORMATION

Use of an automated external defibrillator

An AED can give an electric shock to restart the heart's natural rhythm. AEDs give verbal instructions to the rescuer and are available in many sports clubs, airports, shopping centres and factories. Look for the indication sign in Figure 5.16 (p. 33).

1. Check ABCs
2. Call for help and ask for the AED
3. Commence resuscitation using the ABC method
4. Check for a pulse
5. If there is no pulse, prepare the AED
6. Prepare the athlete by cutting off the shirt, drying the chest. Quickly shaving the chest hair may be required before attaching the AED electrode pads, to give a better contact
7. A second rescuer should continue resuscitation until the AED electrode pads are attached in the positions shown in Figure 5.17 (p. 34). The AED analyses the heart rhythm and will not fire unless it is appropriate
8. **Make sure no one is touching the athlete**
9. **Press the 'shock' button only if directed verbally by the AED**
10. Continue with resuscitation.

Do not leave player unattended while waiting for medical team to arrive.

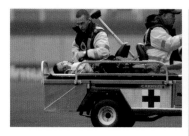

Non-cardiac chest pain

Many people (and most young people) have chest pain that is not caused by the heart – this is called non-cardiac chest pain.

What causes non-cardiac chest pain?

The most common cause of non-cardiac chest pain arises from a nearby organ, the oesophagus.

- Gastro-oesophageal reflux disease (GORD) – back up of stomach acid into the oesophagus causing heartburn and chest pain
- Musculoskeletal problems – muscle inflammation or bruising of the chest wall
- Anxiety – anxiety and panic attacks can produce chest pain that resembles the pain experienced during a heart attack

The diagnosis that chest pain is not related to the heart should only be made by trained medical professionals.

'I CAN'T BREATHE AND I HAVE PAIN IN MY CHEST – I WAS HIT

Red Zone

- **Broken ribs**
- **Collapsed lung**
- **Windpipe injury**

Amber Zone

- Rib/sternal injury

Green zone

- **Winded**

Broken ribs/breast bone (sternum)

Broken ribs (Fig. 15.6) are a common injury in contact sports. They are caused by direct trauma to the ribcage. The player will complain of severe pain with deep breathing and tenderness over the injured area.

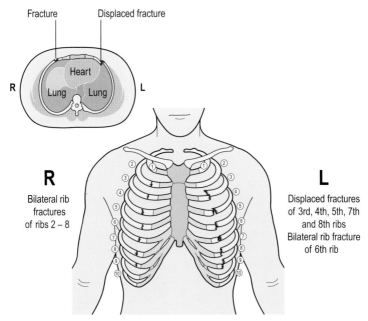

R — Bilateral rib fractures of ribs 2 – 8

L — Displaced fractures of 3rd, 4th, 5th, 7th and 8th ribs. Bilateral rib fracture of 6th rib

Fracture   Displaced fracture

Heart

Lung   Lung

R   L

Fig. 15.6 Broken ribs.

What should I check for?

Speak to the player

- 'What happened?'
- 'Did you get hit?'
- 'Do you have any pain?'
  - 'Point to the pain!'
  - 'Did you hear a crack?'
  - 'Are you having trouble breathing?'
- 'Does it hurt to take a deep breath in?'

Problem identification

- A player who has received a serious blow to the chest will be in some distress
- They may have heard a crack or felt a pop on impact. This would point to a cracked rib, injured breast bone (sternum) or popped cartilage
- The area of the soreness should be easily localized
- A rib injury will typically give increased pain on deep breathing

Observe

- Observe the way the player is breathing
  - Initially, the player may be 'winded' – unable to catch their breath
  - The player may be anxious or in distress
  - The breathing pattern is fast and shallow – not unlike hyperventilation, but the player will have pain!

- Pay attention to the player's ability to speak in sentences. If the player is unable to complete a full sentence they may have injured their lung underneath and have a pneumothorax

- If the player is in severe distress they will be using other muscles to breathe:
  - Sucking in of their cheeks
  - Sucking in of their stomachs
  - Straining of the muscles in their neck

Rule out serious injury

This **is** a serious injury – but be careful to also look out for:

- Pneumothorax (collapsed lung) – the player who has severe shortness of breath; see 'Collapsed lung', below

- Cardiac injury (exceptionally rare) – severe pain behind the breast bone with extreme tenderness on touching (see below)

- Splenic injury (rare) – severe pain on the left side of the abdomen

- Liver injury (rare) – severe pain on the right side of the abdomen

Touch for tenderness

- Feel over the sore area identified by the player for any abnormalities of the ribs

- Feel over the breast bone (sternum): place your fingers on either side of the breast bone and press down – this will be painful if there is any injury to the sternum or ribs

- Expose the skin to look for any bruising, bleeding or deformities. This will also allow you to observe both sides of the chest moving simultaneously

- Feel each side of the chest wall to see if they are moving equally with each breath

- Feel over the airway in the neck to see if it remains in the middle or is moved to one side – usually away from the side of injury. This indicates a collapsed lung and is a severe emergency

Skills assessment

This is not applicable. A player with a fractured rib **must** not continue physical activity as they may cause further damage.

What should I do?

Talk to the player

Act calmly and with assurance – tell the player they are coming off.

Remove the player safely from the field of play

Emergency transfer

A player with a fractured rib should be taken to hospital by whatever means available. **If they have a collapsed lung, they need an ambulance urgently!**

Avoid further injury

- You must remove the player from competition if a rib fracture is suspected

- Stopping activity will reduce the stress on the heart and lungs

Treatment

- Place the player in a seated position

- Monitor their breathing closely: deep breaths will be painful but it is important to try to get the player to calm down their breathing if it is too fast

  - Get the player to breathe slowly with you

  - Count their breaths

- Keep the player warm

- Give oxygen if available

- Place ice over the injured area

- Give pain relief if available

- Any suspicion of a fractured rib requires investigation by a doctor then player should be sent to hospital for an

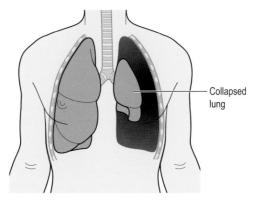

Fig. 15.7 Collapsed lung on the right side.

X-ray to rule out any lung injury

Collapsed lung (pneumothorax)

Pneumothorax (Fig. 15.7) is a collection of air between the outside surface of the lung and the inside surface of the chest wall causing the lung to collapse. Collapsed lung is a rarely encountered injury in sport. It may be caused by blunt trauma to the chest in contact sports or by an accident in motor sports. Symptoms such as shortness of breath and pain with breathing begin immediately after the injury. This is a potentially life-threatening condition for the player and needs to be dealt with urgently by a doctor.

What should I check for?

Speak to the player

- 'What happened?'
- 'Are you having trouble breathing?'
- 'Did you get hit?'
- 'Do you have any pain in the chest?'
- 'Where is the pain?'
- 'Does it hurt to breathe in?'
- 'Has this ever happened before?'

Problem identification

- The player will complain of a sharp pain and localize it to one side of the chest
- They may have felt a crack or heard a pop following impact – this would indicate that a rib or cartilage has been damaged

- The pain is worse on taking a deep breath

- The player will have increasing difficulty talking as the air in the chest cavity expands, reducing the volume of the lung

- The player will become more anxious as their breathing becomes more difficult

Observe

- Observe the way the player is breathing

  - The player could be anxious and in respiratory distress

  - Watch the movement of the rib cage – one side will not move compared to the other

  - Watch to see if the player is using other muscles to breathe – straining of neck muscles, sucking in of the cheeks and tummy as they try to get more air in

  - Look for a bluish tinge to the skin, especially around the lips – this indicates low oxygen levels in the blood

Rule out serious injury

This is a life threatening situation.

- Make sure the airway is open – go immediately to the ABC chapter (p. 21) if the airway closes

- Cardiac injury (exceptionally rare) – severe pain behind the breast bone with extreme tenderness on touching (see below)

- Splenic injury (rare) – severe pain on the left side of the abdomen

- Liver injury (rare) – severe pain on the right side of the abdomen

Touch for tenderness

- Feel over the sore area identified by the player for any abnormalities of the ribs

- Feel over the breast bone (sternum) – place your fingers on either side of the breast bone and press down. This will be painful if there is any injury to the sternum or ribs

- Expose the skin to look for any bruising, bleeding, or deformities. This will also allow you to observe both sides of the chest moving simultaneously

- Feel each side of the chest wall to see if they are moving equally with each breath

- Feel over the airway in the neck to see if it remains in the middle or is moved to one side – usually away from the side of injury. This indicates a collapsed lung and is a severe emergency

Skills assessment
This is not appropriate. The player is not able to continue physical activity.

What should I do?

Talk to the player
Act calmly and with assurance – tension and anxiety make breathing worse.

Remove the player safely from the field of play

Emergency transfer
Call for an ambulance immediately. Explain on the phone that you suspect someone has a pneumothorax.
They may be able to send a doctor to you or trained personnel who can deal with the problem on site.

Avoid further injury

- Stopping activity will reduce the stress on the heart and lungs
- Remove the player from an environment that may cause breathing difficulties – cold, dry, foggy air

Treatment

- Place player in a seated position
- Give oxygen
- Call for medical assistance
- Large collections of air crushing the lungs need

insertion of a chest drain so urgently send patient to the hospital
- A doctor may try to decompress the air in the chest by placing a needle through the chest wall. This should only be carried out by a person with experience

Windpipe injury

A direct injury to the neck damaging the windpipe is life-threatening. Assessing the problem may be difficult if the player cannot speak. Have a very low threshold for sending the player to hospital. This is a very serious emergency. Go to the ABC chapter (p. 21) if in doubt.

What should I check for?

Speak to the player

- 'What happened?'
- 'Did you get hit?'
- 'Do you have any pain?'
  - 'Point to the pain!'
- 'Are you having trouble breathing?'
- 'Does it hurt to take a deep breath in?'

Problem identification

- A player who has received a serious blow to the throat or windpipe will be in some distress

- They may have heard a crack or felt a pop on impact. They will generally grab their throat or neck to protect it
- The area of the soreness should be easily localized
- The player may be able to talk initially, but this can gradually become more difficult as the airway begins to swell

Observe

- Observe the way the player is breathing
  - Initially, the player may be 'winded' – unable to catch their breath
  - The player may be anxious or in distress
  - The breathing pattern is fast and shallow – not unlike hyperventilation, but the player will have pain!
- Pay attention to the player's ability to speak full sentences. If the player is unable to complete a full sentence this may indicate that the airway is closing off. **Go to** the ABC chapter (p. 21)! **Call for an ambulance**!
- If the player is in severe distress they will be using other muscles to breathe:
  - Sucking in of their cheeks
  - Sucking in of their stomachs
  - Straining of the muscles in their neck

Rule out serious injury

This **is** a serious injury – but be careful to also look out for:

- Pneumothorax (collapsed lung) – the player who has severe shortness of breath: refer to 'Collapsed lung' above

Touch for tenderness

- Feel over the sore area identified by the player. Feel over the airway in the neck, down from directly under the chin to where the windpipe enters the chest
- Feel for any deviation of the airway or abnormality – crushed Adam's apple or damaged cartilage in the neck
- Feel over the breast bone (sternum) – place your fingers on either side of the breast bone and press down – this will be painful if there is any injury to the sternum or ribs
- Expose the skin to look for any bruising, bleeding, or deformities. This will also allow you to observe both sides of the chest moving simultaneously
- Feel both sides of the chest wall to see if they are moving equally with each breath

Skills assessment

This is not applicable. A player with an injured windpipe must not continue physical activity as they may cause further damage.

What should I do?

Talk to the player
Act calmly and with assurance
– tell the player they are coming
off.

Remove the player safely from the
field of play

Emergency transfer
**A player with an injured
windpipe should be taken to
hospital immediately by
whatever means are available.**

Avoid further injury
You must remove the player
from the field of play if an
injured or fractured windpipe is
suspected.

Treatment

• Place the player in a seated
position

• Monitor their breathing closely
– deep breaths will be painful,
but it is important to try to get
the player to calm down their
breathing if it is too fast

  • Get the player to breathe
slowly with you

  • Count their breaths

• Keep the player warm

• Give oxygen if available

• Place ice over the injured area

• Give pain relief if available

• Any suspicion of an injured
wind pipe requires
investigation by a doctor and
the player should be sent to
hospital for an X-ray to rule
out any lung injury

Rib/sternal injury or just winded?

It is very difficult to decide
between an injury to the chest
caused by contact that is serious
and not so serious. The key to
making this decision is to speak
to the player and determine how
severe the contact was. A player
who has suffered a serious injury
will not want to play on. It is
important to give the player
plenty of time to recover. If a
bruise or lesser injury is
suspected, it is reasonable to let
the player try to play on.
However, you must watch them
carefully. If they are struggling,
take them off. If a player is just
winded, they'll be able to run it
off after a few minutes.

What should I check for?

Speak to the player

• 'What happened?'

• 'Did you get hit?'

• 'Do you have any pain?'

• 'Point to the pain!'

• 'Are you having trouble
breathing?'

• 'Does it hurt to take a deep
breath in?'

Problem identification

- A player who has received a serious blow to the chest will be in some distress
- They will not have heard a crack or felt a pop on impact
- The area of the soreness should be easily localized
- The player may have increased pain on breathing but this should settle down
- Being winded can be frightening and the player may be quite agitated

Observe

- Observe the way the player is breathing:
  - Initially, the player may be 'winded' – unable to catch their breath
  - The distress will settle quickly if the injury is not severe
  - The breathing pattern is fast and shallow initially but should calm down quickly. The player should not have too much pain!
- The player should be able to speak full sentences with no problem – if they are unable to do this they may have injured their lung underneath and have a pneumothorax
- The player should not be in severe distress or using other muscles to breathe:

- No sucking in of their cheeks
- No sucking in of their stomachs
- No straining of the muscles in their neck

Rule out serious injury
Be careful to also look out for:

- Broken ribs
- Damaged windpipe
- Pneumothorax (collapsed lung) – the player who has severe shortness of breath: refer to 'Collapsed lung' above
- Cardiac injury (exceptionally rare) – severe pain behind the breast bone with extreme tenderness on touching (see below)
- Splenic injury (rare) – severe pain on the left side of the abdomen
- Liver injury (rare) – severe pain on the right side of the abdomen

Touch for tenderness

- Feel over the sore area identified by the player for any abnormalities of the ribs
- Feel over the breast bone (sternum) – place your fingers on either side of the breast bone and press down – **this may be painful with bruised ribs or a bruised sternum**

(Amber Zone Injury); it should not be painful if the player is just winded (Green Zone Injury)

- Expose the skin to look for any bruising, bleeding or deformities. This will also allow you to observe both sides of the chest moving simultaneously

- Feel each side of the chest wall to see if they are moving equally with each breath

- Feel over the airway in the neck to see if it remains in the middle or is moved to one side – usually away from the side of injury – this indicates a collapsed lung and is a severe emergency

Green Zone – Non-painful or very mild pain

Amber Zone –
- **Some pain but not severe**
- **Normal chest movement and breathing**

Skills assessment

- A player who recovers quickly with normal breathing and very minimal pain can play on with close observation

- A player who is tender to touch with delayed recovery or increased effort in breathing should be substituted

- Keep a close eye on any injured player returning to competition. If in doubt, keep them out!

chapter 16

Abdominal injuries

G O Lawlor, G McEntee

INTRODUCTION

Most abdominal injury is due to **blunt trauma**: a punch, headbutt or kick directed at the abdomen in the form of a misdirected tackle or act of aggression. Most blunt trauma is not serious but it can sometimes require a doctor's review.

Penetrating trauma is injury due to actions such as stabbing or shooting, or any injury caused by sharp objects. All require immediate review in a hospital.

Organs in the abdomen can be damaged after blunt or penetrating trauma (Fig. 16.1).

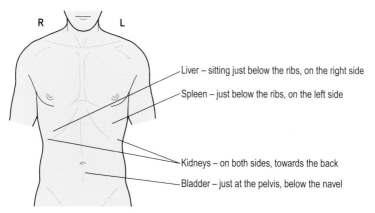

Fig. 16.1 Organs in the abdomen can be damaged after blunt or penetrating trauma.

Deciding on the severity of an injury

- Athlete pale, sweaty, clammy
- Any penetrating trauma
- Severe, unrelenting or worsening abdominal pain with a hard belly
- (In car racing injury) seat belt rash, bruising from steering wheel
- Abdominal bruising
- Unexplained pain of a shoulder tip following injury to the belly
- Severe shortness of breath

These patients require immediate transfer to hospital.

- Mild/moderate belly pain. Athlete is otherwise ok, but winded. **If pain is worse on review later, the athlete's injuries are then in the red zone**
- Vomiting on the field of play is a common occurrence. It could be due to the exercise, perhaps the player just ate, or already had gastroenteritis coming on the pitch, or a blow to the belly upset the stomach. Such injuries stay in the amber zone if symptoms improve over an hour. **The player enters the red zone if they vomit blood, the vomiting worsens, they also had a blow to the head, or they exhibit any red zone symptoms**
- Abdominal wall muscles can be injured by stretching, twisting or a blow to the belly – although this is not serious, it can be difficult to differentiate from serious underlying injury

The athlete should be substituted. Playing on may cause further injury. Review in a short while for any worsening in the injury.

The athlete can return to play if:
- Pain is not severe (rated at less than 6 out of 10)
- Patient is completely alert
- There is no localized tenderness to suggest organ or rib injury

ABDOMINAL INJURY

What should I check for?

Speak to the player

- 'How did the injury happen?'
- 'Where is the pain? Point to the sore area'
- 'How bad is the pain?' (scale of 1 to 10: 1 is no pain, 10 is extreme pain)
- 'Does the pain spread anywhere else?'
- 'Are there any other injuries?'

Problem identification

- A player in a lot of pain will usually not play on!
- Finding the site or cause of the pain is easy. Judging how serious it is is where the difficulty arises

Finding the site or cause of the pain is easy. Judging how serious it is, that's the difficulty!

> ### INSTRUCTION
>
> You won't be criticised for caution! If you are unsure, seek help immediately.

Observe

- Is the athlete breathing normally? Abnormal breathing may indicate serious injury to the muscles of breathing or injury to the spinal cord

- Is the patient alert? Look for signs of faintness or lightheadedness
- Does movement make the pain worse? In serious injury, the patient is unable to move because of the pain (Of course, the contrary is not true. Just because a patient can move doesn't mean there is not a serious underlying injury)
- Vomiting – If the athlete is vomiting, it may be a serious sign of head injury that requires immediate referral to hospital
- Look for deep cuts: shallow cuts can be cleaned and covered with gauze. Deep or gaping cuts require **immediate medical attention** for examination of the wound

Rule out serious injury

- Observe for any of the danger signs – if symptoms or signs are in the red zone (see p. 157), **refer the player directly to hospital**

Touch for tenderness

- Lie the player down, sweater off, flat on their back on the ground, legs flat on the ground and hands down by the sides
- Look for any obvious injuries – cuts/grazes, bruising, masses or swelling
- With the flat part of your fingers, press down gently on the player's abdomen in all areas. (Fig. 16.2)

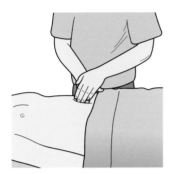

Fig. 16.2 Gently press on different parts of the abdomen.

- Look for areas of focal tenderness caused by the pressure of your hand. Also note any abnormal masses
- **Pay particular attention to any tenderness over the ribs.** A broken rib can lead to further injury – it can tear the liver or spleen

Skills assessment

- Can the player get back to play? See if they can stand up and walk around without much discomfort

What should I check for?

Talk to the player

- Reassure the player, explain what is going on

Remove from the field of play

- Minor injuries may be dealt with on the field of play

- More serious injuries should be assessed on the sideline (**Amber Zone Injury**). With Amber zone injuries, patients who do not need immediate transfer to hospital can be observed. Reassess later for change in condition

Emergency management

- **Transfer the patient immediately to hospital**

Avoid further injury

- Rest the patient, and examine periodically for any changes
- Observe the player who plays on. They may not be able to 'run off' the injury and may need to come off

Treatment

- Call for transport to hospital
- Only sips of fluid – no food or drink until examined by a doctor
- Limit hypothermia by making sure the player is kept warm
- **Athletes in the amber zone may also require medical attention,** although the features are less immediately life-threatening)
- Pain relief with paracetamol only – stronger pain relief will mask important symptoms
- Rest the patient until decision to transfer to hospital is made

Red Zone

- Severe pain (severity >6/10)
- Abnormal swelling or shape of a testicle – compare it to opposite testicle
- Bruising, darkening or swelling of the scrotum

These patients require immediate transfer to hospital. (Note: one testicle hanging lower than the other is normal.)

Amber Zone

- Moderate genital pain. No obvious signs of injury
- Pain improves over an hour

The athlete should be substituted. Playing on may cause further injury. Re-review in a short while for any worsening in the injury.

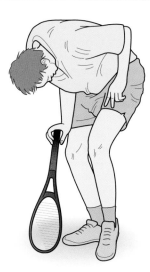

Fig. 16.3 A tennis ball is a common cause of injury to the genital area.

Green Zone

- The pain is not severe (rated at less than 6 out of 10), improving and athlete can play unhindered
- Athlete is completely alert and not vomiting
- There are no obvious abnormalities on examination

The athlete can return to play.

- Sit on sideline for brief observation period if necessary. Pain relief with paracetamol only
- Return to play if pain improves, no worrying features (see p. 158), and player is feeling better

INJURIES TO THE GENITALIA – 'A KICK IN THE BALLS'

This usually occurs as a result of blunt trauma; e.g. kick, punch, golf or tennis ball projectile (Fig. 16.3).

What should I check for?

Speak to the player

- 'How did the injury happen?'
- 'How bad is the pain?' (scale of 1 to 10: 1 is no pain, 10 is extreme pain)

- 'Does the pain spread anywhere else?'

- 'Are there any other injuries?'

Problem identification

- A player in a lot of pain will usually not play on!

- Finding the site or cause of the pain is easy. Judging how serious it is is where the difficulty arises

Observe

- Does movement make the pain worse? In serious injury, the patient is unable to move because of the pain (Of course, the contrary is not true. Just because a patient can move doesn't mean there is not a serious underlying injury)

- Vomiting – Vomiting is common in injuries to the genitals and thus not too worrying – it usually resolves as the pain eases

- Look for deep cuts: shallow cuts can be cleaned and covered with gauze. Deep or gaping cuts require **immediate medical attention** for examination of the wound

Rule out serious injury

- Observe for any of the danger signs – if symptoms or signs are in the red zone (see p. 161), **refer the player directly to hospital**

Touch for tenderness
This is not necessary in minor blows. But if pain is not resolving or there is concern of serious injury, try the following:

- **Males**: With a gloved hand, gently hold each testicle between your thumb and second finger and roll it between your fingers, looking for any obvious abnormal lump or tenderness

- **Females**: Look for any obvious swellings or bleeding

Skills assessment

- Can the player get back to play? See if they can stand up and walk around without much discomfort

What should I do?

Talk to the player

- Reassure the player, explain what is going on

Remove from the field of play

- Minor injuries may be dealt with on the field of play

- More serious injuries should be assessed on the sideline (Amber Zone Injury). With Amber zone injuries, patients who do not need immediate transfer to hospital can be observed. Reassess later for change in condition

Emergency management

- **Transfer the patient immediately to hospital**

Avoid further injury

- Rest the patient, and examine periodically for any changes

- Observe the player who plays on. They may not be able to 'run off' the injury and may need to come off

Treatment

- Call for transport to hospital
- Only sips of fluid – no food or drink until examined by a doctor
- Lie athlete flat on back
- (In males) Ask the player to flex hips and knees. This relieves tension on the scrotum
- Place an ice pack over the genital area
- (In males) elevate the scrotum with the pressure of the ice

pack (if it relieves pain – stop if it worsens pain)

- Pain relief with paracetamol only – stronger pain relief will mask important symptoms

Amber Zone

- **Athletes in the amber zone may also require medical attention,** although the features are less immediately life-threatening)

- As per Red Zone Injury above – ice pack, elevation, pain relief. Observe periodically

Green Zone

- Sit on sideline for brief observation period if necessary
- If necessary, as per Red Zone Injury – ice pack, elevation, pain relief
- Return to play if pain improves fully

Back and pelvis injuries

I Robertson, K Synnott

INTRODUCTION

Back injuries can occur frequently in sport. They can range from minor back strains to severe back injury.

Red Zone

- **Fracture**
- **Bulging disc**
- **Fractured pelvis**

Amber Zone

- Heavy blow to the back
- Back strain/spasm

Green zone

- **Minor blow to the back**

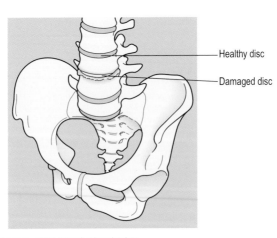

Healthy disc

Damaged disc

Fig. 17.1 Anatomy of the lower back and pelvis.

What should I check for?

Remember SPORTS and do not move the player immediately.

Speak to the player

- 'Where is the pain?'
- 'How severe is the pain?'
- 'Can you move your legs?'

Problem identification

- Identify the extent of the injury by obtaining answers to the questions in the previous section
- For example the player may be complaining of back pain moving down into the back of the leg

Observe

- Do not move the player immediately
- Make sure the player's airway is not compromised
- Look for major abnormalities

Rule out serious injury

- Rule out serious spinal injury
  - Can the player move both legs?
  - Have they full sensation?
  - Are they incontinent of urine or faeces?
- Is there blood coming from the penis/vagina?

Touch for tenderness

- Touch the affected area lightly. Can they feel you touching them?

- Is it very sore to touch?
- Can you feel any abnormalities?

Skills assessment

- If the pain is severe and movement is greatly restricted the player should not continue
- If they have some stiffness but full movement they can play on. Assess at half time and full time

What should I do?

Talk to the player

- Reassure the player and explain what you are doing

Remove from the pitch

- Do not move the player immediately. Trained personnel are essential to protect back and to protect player. See Chapter 7

Emergency transfer

- See Chapter 7

Avoid further injury

- If in any doubt remove player from field of play heeding spinal precautions

Treatment

- If serious injury immobilize on spinal board (Fig. 17.2) and transfer to hospital
- If minor injury apply ice-pack and advise player to rest. Re-assess at half time and full time

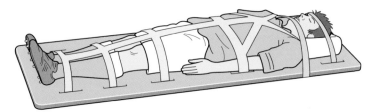

Fig. 17.2 Spinal board immobilization.

Fractured back

What should I check for?

- Severe pain
- Pain moving into back of leg(s)
- No movement of lower limbs
- Decreased/loss of sensation
- Faecal/urinary incontinence

What should I do?

- ABC – see ABC chapter (p. 21)
- Communicate with the player
- Do not move the player
- Apply spinal board – trained personnel essential to protect back and position player
- Compromised airway must be urgently managed
- **Arrange for emergency transfer to hospital**

Bulging disc

What should I look for?

- Severe pain
- Markedly decreased movement of the lower back

- Pain moving into back of limbs
- Loss of sensation
- Incontinence of faeces/urine

What should I do?

- Communicate with the player
- Do not move the player
- Apply spinal board – trained personnel essential to protect back and position player
- Compromised airway must be recognized and urgently managed
- **Arrange for emergency transfer to hospital**

Fractured pelvis

What should I check for?

- Severe pain
- Abnormal shape of pelvis
- Blood coming from penis/vagina

What should I do?

- ABC – see the ABC chapter (p. 21)
- Communicate with the player

- **Do not** loosen clothes/belt around pelvis
- See Chapter 7 for immobilization and transfer
- **Arrange for emergency transfer to hospital**
- **Compromised airway must be urgently managed**

- If pain subsides and player has full range of movement they can resume playing
- Note that minor knocks frequently give rise to increased stiffness as the game goes on. If in doubt, pull them out!

Back strain/spasm, heavy blow to the back/pelvis

What should I check for?

- Moderate pain
- Spasm
- Decreased range of movement

What should I do?

- Talk to and reassure the player
- Remove the player safely from the field of play – spinal board if required
- Apply ice

Minor blow to the back/pelvis

What should I look for?

- Mild pain
- Normal range of motion

What should I do?

- Assess for range of movement and pain
- If full range of movement and pain-free, player can run it off and play on

Green Zone

Table 17.1 Assessing severity of injuries to the back and pelvis

	Pain	Range of movement
Red Zone	+	↓
Amber Zone	−	↓
Amber Zone	+	−
Green Zone	−	−

Lower limb injuries

M J Shelly, I P Kelly

INTRODUCTION

The lower limb is frequently injured during sport. Fortunately, most injuries are minor and the player can play on. However, it is important to recognise the serious injuries and treat them appropriately. We have divided the lower limb into three areas (Fig. 18.1):

- Groin, hip and thigh area
- Knee and leg area
- Foot and ankle area

We will discuss the various problems that can occur in each zone.

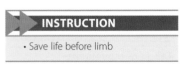

> **INSTRUCTION**
>
> • Save life before limb

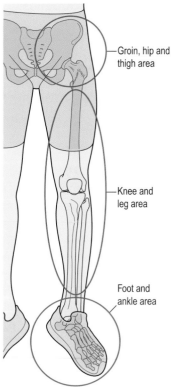

Groin, hip and thigh area

Knee and leg area

Foot and ankle area

Fig. 18.1 The lower limb.

What should I check for?

Speak to the player

- Ensure that the player is conscious and can speak to you in complete sentences (see the ABC chapter (p. 21))

Problem identification

- Ask the player what happened. Get details of the injury:
- 'How did you land?'
- 'Did you feel/hear a crack?' (?Broken bone)
- 'Where is the pain? Point to the sore area'
- 'Does the pain go anywhere or does it stay in the same place?'
- 'Has anything like this happened before?'

Observe

- Is the lower limb obviously deformed? (?Broken bone)
- Is the player holding their leg in a particular way?
- Is there any swelling of the limb? (?Sprained ankle/ twisted knee)
- Is there any obvious bleeding?
- Compare to the opposite limb

Rule out serious injury

Remember – pain in the legs can come from a back injury.

- Can you move your legs? (If not, this indicates a potential back injury: see Ch. 7)

- Any strange sensation/ numbness in the legs? (If yes, treat as a back injury)
- Can you see bone sticking out through the skin? **(Red Zone Injury)**
- Can you see blood spurting out from a wound? **(Red Zone Injury)**

Touch for tenderness
Always wear protective gloves.

- Feel the injured/painful area
- Is it swollen? Is it very sore to touch? (Does the player wince?)
- Can you feel anything broken or unusual?

Skills assessment

- Get the player to move the affected limb
- Get the player to stand up and put weight on sore leg
- If player is unable to bear weight on injured leg (Amber Zone Injury), remove from field immediately and continue assessment on sideline
- Get player to walk/run a few metres – watch for a limp

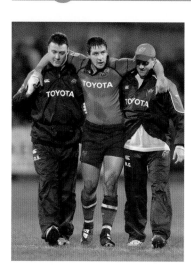

GROIN, HIP AND THIGH

The groin covers the area between the abdomen and the thigh. Serious injuries to the hip are rare, but must be dealt with quickly and efficiently. The thigh is a commonly injured area and injuries here can lead to a player being substituted.

Red Zone

- **Broken hip bones**
- **Hip dislocation**
- **Broken thigh bone**

Amber Zone

- Groin strain
- Hamstring tear
- 'Dead leg' (severely bruised thigh muscles)

Green zone

- **Muscle cramp**
- **Blow to the hip bones (hip pointer)**
- **Pain in pubic area (osteitis pubis)**
- **Minor muscle strains/bruised thigh muscles**

Broken hip/dislocated hip/ broken thigh bone

This can occur suddenly. It is usually the result of a very forceful blow to the hip or a fall from a height.

What should I check for?

- The player will complain of severe pain in the hip or thigh
- The player's leg on the injured side may be shortened – rolled out to the side
- The player will not be able to put weight on the injured leg
- It will be extremely sore when the leg is moved

What should I do?

Talk to the player

- Reassure the player

Remove from the field of play

- Remove the player from the field on a stretcher, with the legs in a splint. See Chapter 10

Emergency transfer to hospital

Avoid further injury

- Do not bend the leg – if it is painful to weightbear, the player should be lifted

Treatment

- Splint
- Rest/Ice/Compression/ Elevation/Diagnosis (RICED – see Fig. 9.5, p. 63)

What should I check for?

Speak to the player

- Reassure the player
- 'What happened?'
- 'Are you in pain?'
- 'Did you hear/feel a crack?'

Problem identification

- Identifying the problem should be obvious. The player will point to the injured hip/thigh
- The player will be in severe pain
- The player may have heard or felt a snap or crack

- The player may have felt the hip pop out

Observe

- The injured leg may appear shortened or rotated outwards (broken hip; Fig. 18.2)
- The injured leg may appear shortened, bent or rotated inwards (dislocated hip; Fig. 18.3)
- Compare the leg to the opposite side
- There may be swelling or deformity

Rule out serious injury

- Ensure that the player is conscious; if not, go to the ABC chapter (p. 21)
- Make sure the player can move the opposite leg and has normal feeling – rule out a spinal injury
- **Pain in the leg may come from the back**

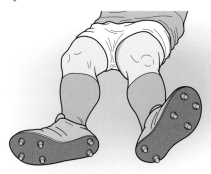

Fig. 18.2 Broken right hip – leg is shortened on left and rolled outwards.

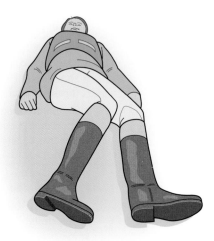

Fig. 18.3 Dislocated right hip – leg is rolled inwards.

Touch

- Ask the player to gently bend up their hip
- Gently roll the injured leg from side to side at the ankle
- If the hip is broken, this will be painful
- Feel over the hip for tenderness

Skills assessment

- If the above tests are not painful, ask the player to stand up
- Place the injured leg on the ground. The player will not be able to weightbear

What should I do?

Talk to the player

- Reassure the athlete, explain what is happening

Remove the player safely from the field of play

- If a neck injury is suspected, the player should have spine and back stabilization prior to transfer
- If there are minor injuries to the leg, the player should be supported off
- If there are major injuries (e.g. broken bone) a stretcher is needed)

Emergency transfer to hospital

- Any neck or spine injuries
  – ambulance

- Broken bones/dislocation
  – quickest possible means

Avoid further injury

- Immobilize the injured leg

- Ensure no neck injury or other injury

- **Any player who cannot perform basic skills runs the risk of doing more damage and should not continue**

Treatment

- Immobilization techniques

- Application of ice

- Application of compressive bandage (if necessary)

- Administration of painkillers (by trained personnel only)

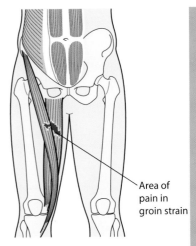

Fig. 18.4 Area of pain in groin strain.

Area of pain in groin strain

What should I check for?

- Player will 'pull up' while running – might have a painful limp

- Player will complain of pain in the groin (Fig. 18.4)

- There will be tenderness in the upper inner thigh

What should I do?

- Ask player to walk/run a few metres – try and gauge whether the player can continue

- This player is unlikely to continue – substitute and apply ice to affected groin (RICE principle – see Fig. 9.6, p. 64)

- Refer for specialist assessment and opinion

- Remove player from the field

- Player must be fully assessed on the sideline to decide whether he/she can return to play or needs to be substituted

Groin strain

Very common injury, especially in soccer.

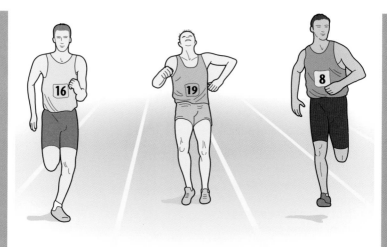

Fig. 18.5 Athlete 'pulls up' with hamstring injury.

Hamstring tears

These are very common injuries that occur suddenly while a player is running/straining. The player commonly 'pulls up' and starts to limp.

What should I check for?

- Player will 'pull up' while running (Fig. 18.5) – may have a painful limp. A hamstring tear feels like being shot in the back of the leg
- Player will complain of pain and swelling behind knee

What should I do?

- Get player to run a few metres – if severe pain – substitute player
- Apply ice to affected area (RICE principle)
- Refer for specialist assessment and treatment

Severe thigh muscle bruise – 'dead leg'/'dead backside'

This is a very common injury. It is very painful and frequently prevents a player continuing in a game. It is caused by a direct blow to the thigh (Fig. 18.6).

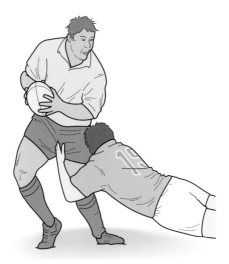

Fig. 18.6 'Dead leg' after a direct blow to the thigh.

What should I check for?

- Player will complain of pain in the affected thigh
- There may be swelling and evidence of bruising
- The muscle commonly feels very hard and painful to touch

What should I do?

- Ask player to walk/run a few meters
- Rub affected area and apply cold spray
- The player may try to run it off. Observe closely
- If unable to continue – apply ice to affected area (RICE principle)
- Refer for specialist assessment and treatment

These are the most common type of sports injury. The vast majority are minor and do not require the player to leave the field of play. If a player is in a lot of pain, substitute and reassess later.

Muscle cramp

Very common, especially near the end of a very strenuous game on a hot day.

Green zone

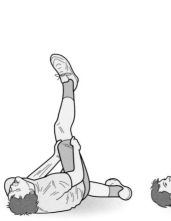 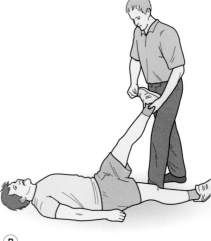

Fig. 18.7 (A) Muscle cramp (B) On-field stretching of muscles to relieve cramp.

What should I check for?

- Player will complain of severe pain in the affected thigh without any impact. The pain will be crampy – like a knot in the muscle

- Player will be unable to continue running – may be unable to remain standing

- Player will have a painful limp on the affected side

What should I do?

- Get player to lie down on ground

- Stretch affected muscles (Fig. 18.7)

- If unable to continue – substitute and allow to rest. No further treatment is necessary

Hip bone bruising

A common injury in contact sports caused by the player receiving a blow over the bony part of the hip (Fig. 18.8). It can be very painful but it does not prevent the player from continuing activity.

What should I check for?

- Player will complain of pain over the bony part of the hip

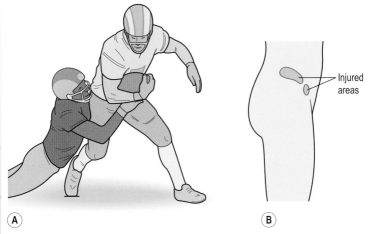

Injured areas

Fig. 18.8 (A) Bruising caused by direct blow to hip (B) injured areas.

- Feel the painful area: if it is very painful, substitute player

What should I do?

- Get player to walk/run a few metres – assess whether he/she can continue
- If pain is slight – allow player to continue and reassess later

Pain in pubic area/kick to 'the privates'

See also Chapter 16.

This occurs after a direct impact to the genital area. Obviously in males, the genitalia are more vulnerable; however, females may also require assessment and treatment.

The player may be breathless with the severity of the pain. They are usually writhing around in pain holding the affected area.

What should I check for?

Talk to the player

- 'Where are you sore?'
- 'Can you feel two testicles?'
- 'Do they feel normal?'
- 'Is the penis or scrotum injured or bleeding?'

What should I do?

- Encourage the male player to support the sore area with both hands. Bending up his knees to the chest may help
- If the pain fully settles and the player feels fine, he can usually resume play
- If the pain persists, remove the player for an appropriate examination by trained personnel in an appropriate environment
- Any bruising, swelling, bleeding or persistent pain needs specialist review

Minor muscle strains/ bruised thigh muscles

Very common injuries. The vast majority are minor and will not prevent a player from continuing.

What should I check for?

- Player will complain of pain in the affected thigh
- There may be swelling and evidence of bruising

What should I do?

- Ask player to walk/run a few metres
- If pain-free/pain settles, allow player to play on

See Chapter 9.

KNEE AND LEG AREA

The knee joint is very commonly injured in sport. The majority of injuries are to the ligaments and muscles, not bone. The leg is injured less commonly than the knee, but injuries here can prevent a player continuing in a game.

Red Zone

- **Broken leg**
- **Twisted knee**
- **Dislocated knee cap**

Amber Zone

- **Swollen knee**
- **Torn calf muscle**
- **Shin splints**

Green zone

- **Bruising of calf muscle**
- **Muscle cramp**

Serious injuries of the knee can occur and must be dealt with quickly and efficiently so that serious damage can be minimized. Broken bones in the leg are not uncommon and simple on-field measures can reduce pain and prevent serious complications.

If you think that a player has a Red Zone injury they must be safely removed from the field of play and transferred to hospital as soon as possible.

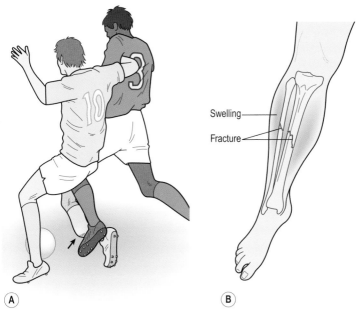

Fig. 18.9 (A) Broken leg from a tackle (B) the bones involved.

Broken leg

This type of injury is common in contact sports and motor sport (Fig. 18.9). It is the result of a direct blow to the leg or an awkward landing after a jump.

What should I check for?

- Player will complain of severe pain in the injured leg
- The player may have heard or felt a snap
- The leg may be obviously deformed – be careful: the leg can be broken without obvious deformity
- The leg may be swollen
- Look for a wound – can you can see bone/blood spurting/ deep cut in the skin?

What should I do?

- **Call an ambulance**
- If bone visible in wound – cover with sterile dressing (if available)
- If blood spurting from wound – apply firm pressure with sterile dressing, putting

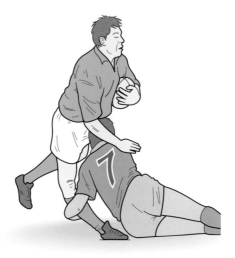

Fig. 18.10 Twisted knee – a serious injury.

enough pressure on to stop the bleeding

- Apply a splint to the affected leg – this will relieve pain (see Fig. 10.2, p. 72)
- Carefully remove player from field on a stretcher

Twisted knee

This is a very serious injury that can have serious consequences for the injured player (Fig. 18.10). The knee relies on ligaments and muscles for stability. If these are torn, the knee becomes very painful and swollen. In the long term, recovery can be slow and incomplete.

What should I check for?

Speak to the player

- 'What happened?'
- 'Where does it hurt?'
- 'How did you fall?'
- 'Did you hear a 'pop' in your knee?'
- 'Did you feel the knee give way under you?'

Observe

- Look for swelling – if knee swells up quickly **it is a Red Zone injury**

Touch

- Touch the knee – is it extremely painful? If yes **it is a Red Zone injury**

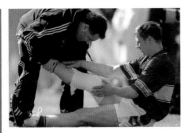

Skills assessment

Ask player to weight bear on affected knee. If unable to, remove from field immediately and reassess on sideline.

What should I do?

- Remove player from field
- Apply support dressing and ice (RICE principle – reduces swelling)
- Give pain killers (if available)
- Transfer to hospital for further assessment

Dislocated kneecap

This can occur suddenly in someone who has had a previous dislocation, or it can happen in a previously normal person as a result of a direct blow to the knee cap

What should I check for?

- The player will complain of pain in the affected knee cap
- The position of the knee cap when compared to the opposite knee may look abnormal (Fig. 18.11)

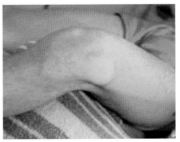

Fig. 18.11 Dislocated knee cap.

Remember – the knee cap can relocate immediately after injury.

- Ask the player if they felt or saw their knee cap dislocate
- Look for any obvious swelling/wounds
- Is the leg deformed – can the player straighten the leg fully?

What should I do?

- Remove player from field
- Apply compression dressing and ice (RICE)
- Trained personnel can 'pop' the kneecap back in place
- Transfer to hospital for further assessment

Amber Zone injuries of the leg and knee are not as serious as Red Zone injuries, but they can be very painful and will usually prevent a player from continuing in the game.

Swollen knee

This is a common injury in all forms of sport but particularly

Amber Zone

so in contact sports. Players frequently receive blows to the knee that do not immediately cause discomfort but as the game progresses the pain may increase in severity.

What should I check for?

- Look for swelling/bruising of affected knee – always compare to opposite knee (Fig. 18.12)
- Feel for tenderness. If player is particularly sore in one spot,

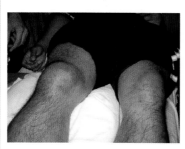

Fig. 18.12 Swollen and bruised knee.

be aware of possible ligament injury – remove player from field

- Can the player put weight on the affected knee? If not, remove player from field for further assessment later

What should I do?

- Get player to put weight on affected knee
- Get player to run/walk a few metres
- Use pain killing 'cold spray'
- Apply compression dressing to knee if pain does not quickly resolve – consider removing player from field

Torn calf muscle/ Achilles tendon

This is similar to a hamstring tear (Fig. 18.13). It usually affects

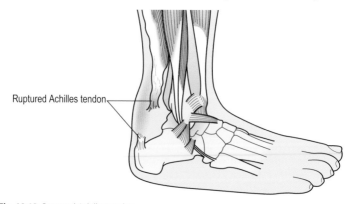

Ruptured Achilles tendon

Fig. 18.13 Ruptured Achilles tendon.

players while they are running and may cause them to pull up. Can be very painful.

What should I check for?

- Look for obvious swelling of calf muscles
- Ask the player where exactly the pain is
- Ask the player to put weight on the affected leg
- Ask the player if they heard a 'snap' when the pain started (if a snap was heard – ?Achilles tendon torn)
- Feel the Achilles tendon on the affected side (compare with other side)

What should I do?

- Remove player from field of play
- If player can weight bear and the Achilles tendon is intact, ask player to run/walk a few metres – consider allowing player to return to play
- If player in severe pain and/or ?Achilles tendon torn – remove player from field and reassess later
- Apply compression bandage and ice (RICE)

Shin splints

This is a general term used to cover the causes of shin pain,

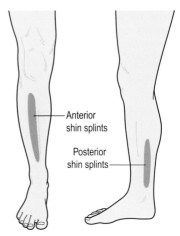

Fig. 18.14 Sites of shin splint pain.

Anterior shin splints

Posterior shin splints

especially pain at the front of the shin (Fig. 18.14). The injured player may have a history of long-term shin pain that has gradually increased in severity over the previous few weeks. The pain occurs with exercise and can become so severe as to prevent the player continuing in the game.

What should I check for?

- Ask the player if they have noticed this type of pain before
- Ask if this pain occurs when the player is at rest or only when exercising (if pain only occurs with exercise – shin splints likely)

- Ask the player if they have increased their level of training recently
- Get the player to put weight on the affected limb
- Feel the shin: if the bone or muscle is painful to touch – think shin splints

What should I do?

- Remove player from field of play for further assessment
- Apply ice – avoid compression bandage
- Get player to run/walk a few metres – if pain intensifies – tell the player to rest, ice and elevate his/her limb
- Refer player for specialist assessment and treatment

What should I check for?

- Player will complain of pain and tenderness over his/her calf muscle
- Some bruising may be evident (Fig. 18.15)
- Get player to walk/run a few metres – if pain improves, player can return to game

What should I do?

- Apply some cold spray to area to provide pain relief

These injuries are very common and frequently occur during the course of sport. They are usually only minor issues that resolve quickly with little or no treatment.

Bruising of calf muscle

Can occur when a player receives a blow to the leg during a match. Initially the injury can be painful but most players are easily able to 'run it off'.

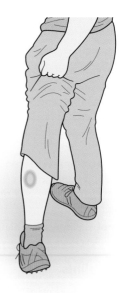

Fig. 18.15 Bruised calf.

Muscle cramp

Very common, especially near the end of a very strenuous game on a hot day.

What should I check for?

- Player will complain of severe pain in the affected leg without any impact. The pain will be crampy – like a knot in the muscle
- Player will be unable to continue running – may be unable to remain standing
- Player will have a painful limp on the affected side

What should I do?

- Get player to lie down on ground
- Stretch affected muscles
- If unable to continue – substitute and allow to rest. No further treatment is necessary

FOOT AND ANKLE AREA

Injuries of the foot and ankle are commonplace in sport. The vast majority are minor and require little more than rest and ice. The ankle is the most commonly injured joint in sport. It is placed under tremendous strain during physical activity. Under certain conditions the very strong ligaments holding the ankle bones together can tear, leading to an ankle sprain or more seriously, a broken ankle. The foot is less frequently injured than the ankle, but injuries here are related to the large stresses placed on the foot during running.

Red Zone

- **Broken ankle**
- **Broken bones in the foot**

Amber Zone

- Ankle sprain
- **Stress fractures of bones in foot**

Green zone

- **Heel pain**
- **Skin blisters**

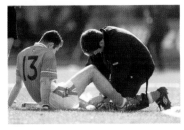

Broken bones in the foot and ankle occur particularly in athletics and sports in which the stresses on the ankle and foot are great, such as tennis. They prevent the player continuing and can lead to long period 'on the bench' as recovery is often long and difficult.

Red Zone

Broken ankle

It is important to be able to tell the difference between a broken ankle and an ankle that is badly sprained. A player with a broken ankle will be in severe pain and will not be able to stand on the affected ankle. The ankle will also swell up quickly.

What should I check for?

- Ask the player how the injury happened – commonly, the player will tell you that they 'went over' on the ankle (Fig. 18.16)
- Look for swelling/bruising/ deformity of the ankle (there may be a lot!!)
- Ask the player to stand on the affected ankle – if they refuse to attempt to do so or are unable to do so – **red flag** – suspect a broken ankle

What should I do?

- Apply ice and splint/elevate foot (RICE)
- Remove player from field of play
- Give painkillers (if available)
- **Call an ambulance to transfer player to hospital**

Note for doctor: If ankle is very deformed – relocate as soon as possible.

Broken bone in the foot

This is usually due to repeated stress to a bone in the foot (Fig. 18.17) but it can occur suddenly as a result of a direct blow to the foot from a tackle.

What should I check for?

- Ask the player how the injury happened
- Ask the player where the pain is located – the painful area will be quite specific
- Look for any swelling or bruising over the painful area
- Ask the player to stand on the affected foot – if unable to weightbear – **red flag** – broken bone in foot

What should I do?

- Remove player from field of play
- Apply ice and elevate foot
- **Transfer to hospital as soon as possible**

Ankle sprains are less serious than a broken ankle but can be nasty injuries. If you suspect someone has an ankle sprain, remove them from the field of play. Stress fractures of the bones of the foot can cause

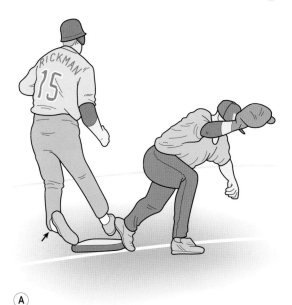

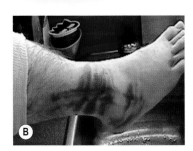

Fig. 18.16 (A) Twisting injury that leads to broken ankle. (B) Bruising and swelling associated with a broken ankle.

chronic, annoying pain that only occurs with exercise. The danger is that a small stress break in the bone may become a full break if the player puts the bone under too much stress.

Ankle sprains

Ankle sprains (Fig. 18.18) can be difficult to tell apart from a broken ankle. Both are painful, both will cause the ankle to swell

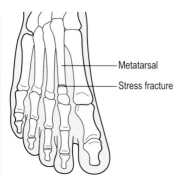

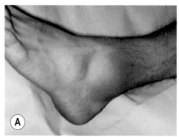

Fig. 18.17 Stress fracture of a bone in the foot.

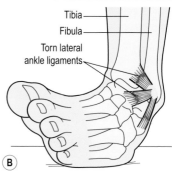

Fig. 18.18 (A) Sprained ankle. (B) Some of the ligaments that commonly tear.

and be bruised. The major difference between them is that a broken ankle, as a general rule, will have **more** pain, **more** swelling and **more** bruising than a sprained ankle. A player should be able to stand on a sprained ankle (unless it is very badly sprained) but not on a broken ankle.

What should I check for?

- Ask the player what happened
- Ask where the pain is – get the player to point to the painful spot (frequently, one side of the ankle hurts more than the other)
- Look for swelling and bruising (not as evident as in a broken ankle)
- Ask the player to stand on the affected ankle

What should I do?

- Remove the player from the field of play
- Apply a compression bandage, ice and elevate (RICE)
- If no improvement in symptoms – refer for specialist opinion

Stress fracture of bone in foot

This is less serious than a broken bone in the foot, but it can be very painful and stop the player from continuing in the game.

What should I check for?

- Ask the player how the injury happened. Have they had this pain before?
- Ask the player where the pain is located – the painful area will be quite specific
- Look for any swelling or bruising over the painful area
- The player should be able to stand on the foot, but it may be very painful

What should I do?

- Remove player from field of play
- Apply ice and elevate foot
- If pain does not settle over a period of hours – transfer hospital for further assessment

Minor injuries to the foot and ankle are common. Skin blisters can cause significant discomfort and prevent a player from competing. Heel pain can be caused by many different things, but the vast majority are due to overuse/overtraining and respond to simple measures such as rest and physiotherapy.

Heel pain

The Achilles tendon can become inflamed where it attaches to the bones in the foot. Pain is usually gradual in onset and can be associated with a new training regime or even new footwear. Pain occurs with exercise and remains as an ache when the player is at rest.

What should I check for?

- Player will complain of a nagging pain that gets worse with exercise and remains when at rest
- Ask about new footwear/ training regimes
- Look for swelling/bruising over the Achilles tendon
- Feel for tenderness over the heel – it can be in a quite specific area (Fig. 18.19)

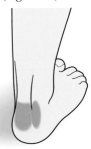

Fig. 18.19 Area where heel pain is most common.

- Get the player to walk/run a few metres: if pain is tolerable, allow player to return to game. If pain gets worse, remove player from field of play

What should I do?

- Apply cold spray to area (provides pain relief)
- If pain recurs, refer player for specialist assessment and treatment

Skin blisters (see Chapter 8)

Blisters on around the foot and ankle are very common, especially after long matches on hard ground or if the player's footwear does not fit correctly. They are very painful and commonly prevent a player from continuing in a game.

What should I check for?

- The player will be walking with a painful limp
- Ask the player to remove their footwear
- Look for evidence of skin blisters (Fig. 18.20)

What should I do?

- Burst the blisters and apply a sterile dressing to the area
- Apply second skin or dressing
- Ask the player to walk/run a few metres: if pain improves, allow player to return to play

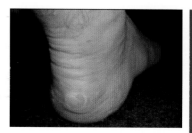

Fig. 18.20 A large heel blister.

– if not, substitute and reassess later

Toenail injuries

These injuries are common in contact sports where studs (cleats) are worn by the participants. They also occur in endurance sports, e.g., marathons.

There is bleeding, which is trapped under the toenail.

What should I check for?

- The player will complain of throbbing pain
- The nail will be discoloured from the underlying blood and may feel loose

What should I do?

- Occasionally, strapping the toe with adhesive tape may allow the player to continue
- Trained personnel will relieve the pressure under the nail by burning a hole in the nail with a heated sterile needle

19

Drowning and water sports injuries

G Horgan, G C O'Toole

DROWNING

500 people drown every day worldwide. Three times as many people go to hospital with near-drowning injuries, which can cause serious brain damage and long-term disability.

Everyone who uses water for recreational purposes and who lives near water should be taught to swim by a qualified instructor.

What do I do if I see someone drowning?

'Personal safety first.' You must have a good grasp on land. You must be able to swim competently yourself if attempting rescue by boat.

The rules for rescuing someone who is drowning are Reach, Throw, Row, Don't go (Fig. 19.1).

INFORMATION

Safety instructions

- Never swim alone and swim near a lifeguard tower
- Check with lifeguards about conditions before swimming
- Don't overestimate your ability
- Wear sunscreen
- Avoid alcohol
- Never run and dive into the sea. You never know how deep it is!
- If you want to swim long distances swim parallel to the shore in your depth
- If you get in trouble try not to panic. Raise your arm for help, float and wait for help to arrive
- If caught in a 'rip' current dragging you out to sea don't fight it. Swim parallel to shore until free of out-rushing water. Now swim back to shore or raise your arm and signal for assistance.
- Stay calm and conserve your energy. If you become tired, float with the current and signal for help.

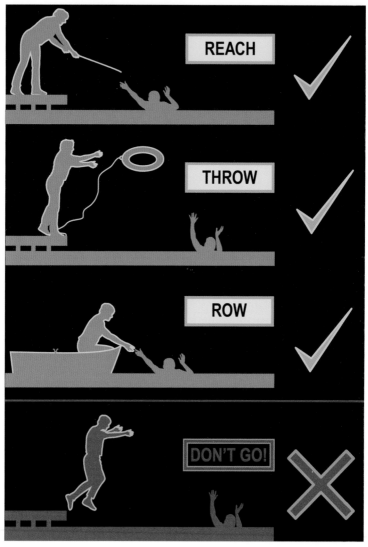

Fig. 19.1 Reach, Throw, Row, Don't go.

Reach

Hold on to the dock or boat and reach your hand, fishing pole, boat oar or whatever you have nearby to the person in trouble in the water.

Throw

If you can't reach far enough, throw objects that will float for the person to hang on to, e.g. ideally a life preserver but plastic bottles, cushions, pieces of wood, plastic picnic containers or anything else that floats.

Row

If you're in a boat, move the boat closer to the person in the water and call to nearby vessels for help.

Don't go

- Stay out of the water unless trained the way lifeguards are trained to rescue injured and frightened people
- Call local emergency number, stay calm and give exact location

How do I safely remove someone from the water?

This is illustrated in Figures 19.2 and 19.3.

What should I do when back on land?

- Bystanders should call emergency services immediately

- **ABC s are priority** (see the ABC chapter, p. 21)

- Remove foreign bodies using jaw thrust manoeuvre

- Rescue breaths may be difficult because of spasm of the larynx/voicebox

- The Heimlich manoeuvre is of no use

- Give 100% oxygen if available

- Remove clothes and wrap in warm blankets

- **Do not stop cardiopulmonary resuscitation (CPR) until arrival in hospital** as hypothermia (cold body temperature) has a protective effect

- **Transfer urgently to nearest hospital**

 INFORMATION

Did you know?

A 2$\frac{1}{2}$-year-old girl submerged for 66 minutes in cold water recovered fully after a long and successful episode of CPR.

People who nearly drown and seem OK are not OK!

- Bystanders should call emergency services immediately

- Give 100% oxygen if available

- Remove clothes and wrap in warm blankets

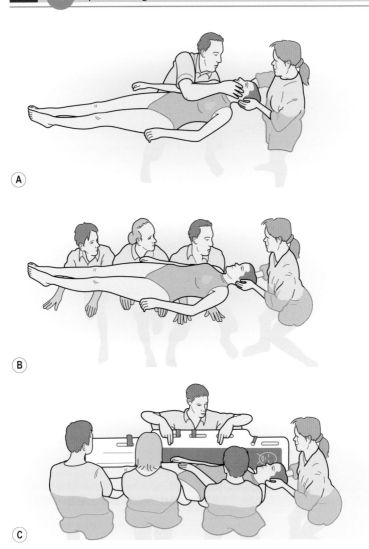

Fig. 19.2 How to remove someone safely from the water. (A) Place the swimmer on to their back Hold the chin and neck steady while getting an assistant to support the head. (B) You will need two further assistants to support the trunk and legs, keeping the back and spine straight. (C) If a spinal board is available, place the board under the swimmer while holding the head and back steady. The swimmer is strapped to the board and brought to shore.

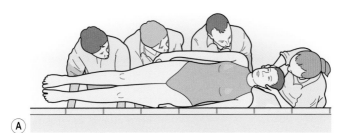

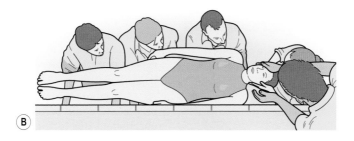

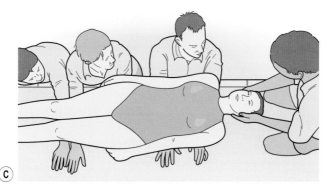

Fig. 19.3 If there is no board available, the swimmer is brought to shore by floating them across the water (A), holding the spine and neck steady at all times. (B) Having reached the shore, a further assistant is needed on shore to hold the head. (C) Ready to move, and move. . . . The swimmer is lifted on to the shore smoothly.

- Transfer to nearest emergency department
- Individuals will be kept in hospital for at least 24 hours, as serious lung disease and multiorgan failure can develop shortly after the episode and they can die

DIVING AND OTHER EMERGENCIES THAT CAN OCCUR WHILE SWIMMING

- Neck injuries are common while diving in shallow water

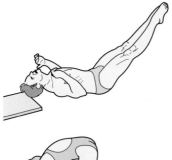

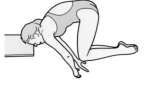

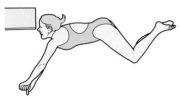

Fig. 19.4 Diving board accidents.

- Remove the person carefully from the water as outlined above
- Once out of the water refer to Chapter 13 on how to evaluate and treat these injuries
- People who swim can have heart attacks or strokes or develop any medical emergency as they would on land – treatment for such people are safe removal from water, ABCs, oxygen and immediate transfer to the nearest emergency department (Fig. 19.5)
- As a special precaution, people who could become unconscious due to, for example, an epileptic seizure or diabetics prone to low blood sugar should never swim as they unnecessarily endanger themselves and others

SCUBA DIVING INJURIES

Before you go

- Arrange an appointment to see a doctor who has an interest in divers as people with medical conditions – e.g. epilepsy, strokes, lung diseases, ear conditions, heart disease and pregnancy – may be at severe risk!

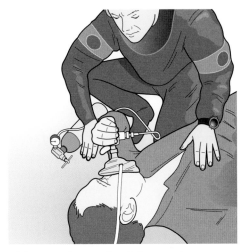

Fig. 19.5 Diver receiving oxygen therapy and medical assessment.

- We recommend learning to dive with a recognized diving school affiliated to the Professional Association of Diving Instructors (PADI). More information about diving courses and physical requirements can be found at www.padi.com
- **Never dive alone**

Problems descending

- The most common injury is damage to the eardrums and middle ear – 'squeeze injuries'
- If someone develops pain in the ear they should signal to their instructor and return safely to the surface under the instructor's direction

- If the pain resolves quickly avoid diving for 2–7 days
- If it persists the person should go to a doctor as severe permanent damage to hearing and balance may occur
- Sometimes water can get into the inner ear and the diver will suddenly lose balance and hearing. This is very frightening and the important thing is to stay calm and signal to the instructor and return safely to the surface. These people need to see a doctor immediately to get treatment for this

Problems at the bottom

- Only touch what instructors signal is safe to touch as there

Red Zone

are many dangerous and poisonous living things in the sea

- If you feel dizzy, disorientated or drunk, signal 'Help!' to the instructor, as the air supply may be malfunctioning

Problems ascending and on the surface

Collapsed lung, gas embolism and decompression sickness are the most common life-threatening emergencies that develop on returning to the surface

- **Collapsed lung** – Failing to exhale on ascent can lead to air expanding and rupture of part of the lung, causing a collapsed lung
- **Gas embolism** – This is when air gets into the circulation because of a small rupture of the lungs. The symptoms develop shortly after resurfacing and there is often a history of an uncontrolled ascent during the dive
- **Decompression sickness ('the bends')** – Too rapid an ascent from a dive may result in nitrogen accumulating throughout the body, forming bubbles. It can take 24 hours to develop but most cases occur in the first 8 hours

Safe removal from water and assessment of ABCs are the priority. If someone has experienced difficulty during the dive or in the 24 hours after the dive, assess the diver with **SPORTS** and **TREAT**.

What should I check for?

Speak to the diver
Check for the following symptoms:

- Chest pain or tightness
- Shortness of breath and coughing
- Numbness, weakness, sensory changes, light-headedness or personality changes
- Loss of balance and hearing
- Severe abdominal pain, vomiting and nausea
- Unexplained joint and muscle pain

Problem identification
If the patient complains of any of the above symptoms one must assume they have developed either, a collapsed lung, gas embolism or decompression sickness as outlined above.

Observe
If the diver feels fine but has froth in the mouth or nose, blotching of the skin or change in personality or behaviour, you must assume that they have

developed one of the above three conditions.

Rule out serious injury

A quick head-to-toe assessment looking for trauma, bites, puncture wounds, jellyfish stings, etc. must be performed.

Touch

- Examine the patient's ABCs regularly and administer CPR if necessary

- Touch the joints and abdomen and, if there is severe pain, assume that the diver has decompression sickness

- If a patient develops a collapsed lung they may have a swollen neck or chest due to air trapped under the skin. This feels like a crackling sensation when you touch the skin. The next step is to give 100% oxygen and to examine the chest as outlined in Chapter 12. If the diver is very short of breath one must consider inserting a chest needle through the rib cage to relieve the collapsed lung, as explained in Chapter 15

Skills assessment

Under no circumstances should a diver with any of the above features go back in the water or try to be recompressed by diving again.

What should I do?

- **T**alk to the diver and try to calm them down

- **R**emove the diver from the water safely as outlined above if in difficulty

- Emergency transfer – the diver must be transferred urgently to the nearest emergency department, preferably one with a hyperbaric chamber

- **A**void further injury by not letting the diver back in the water under any circumstances

- **T**reat the diver by lying them flat on their back, CPR if necessary, give 100% oxygen if available and wrap them in warm blankets to prevent hypothermia. Wounds and injuries to limbs should be treated as in the appropriate chapter

On the mountain

J M Queally, D McCormack

INTRODUCTION

More and more people are visiting high altitude areas (Fig. 20.1) while skiing, trekking, mountaineering or even visiting a city at altitude (e.g. La Paz in Bolivia at 4200 m). Altitude sickness can range from simple fatigue to life-threatening coma. It is related to individual physiology (genetics) and the

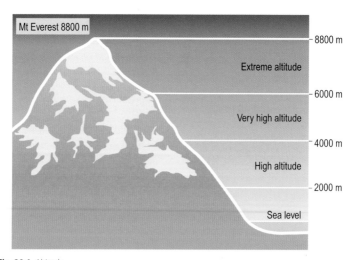

Mt Everest 8800 m

8800 m

Extreme altitude

6000 m

Very high altitude

4000 m

High altitude

2000 m

Sea level

Fig. 20.1 Altitude.

rate of ascent, and not to age, gender, physical fitness or previous altitude experience.

This chapter shows how to recognize and treat the various forms of altitude illness. Acute mountain sickness is the most common form of altitude illness experienced. Treatment often involves simple actions such as rest or descent. However at more extreme altitudes where severe forms of altitude illness are more likely to occur, treatment is often difficult as medical resources are usually limited.

What is high altitude?

- High altitude is defined by scale (Fig. 20.2)
- Practically speaking, altitude illness rarely occurs below 2500 m

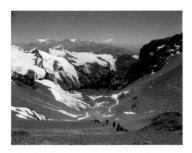

Fig. 20.2 Panoramic views are great but altitude needs to be treated with respect.

Acclimatization

Acclimatization is the normal physiological process of the body adjusting to the decreased availability of oxygen at high altitudes. The body recognizes that oxygen is in short supply and takes a number of steps to increase the amount of oxygen taken in, and more importantly to use that oxygen more efficiently than normal. As you ascend, each breath contains less and less oxygen. To compensate for this lack of oxygen, breaths taken are deeper and more frequent, particularly on exertion (e.g. trekking). This is normal and an important mechanism in adapting to the lack of oxygen. Occasionally 'periodic breathing' can occur, particularly at night. This consists of cycles of normal breathing that gradually slow to a period of not breathing for up to 15 seconds. This is then followed by a brief recovery phase of rapid breathing. Even though this may cause anxiety, it is important to realize that this is not altitude sickness but rather a manifestation of the normal acclimatization process. Rates of acclimatization differ between individuals. After 10 days at altitude the body is approximately 80% acclimatized for most people.

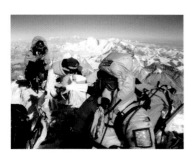

Fig. 20.3 Above 8000 m even acclimatization is not enough. Supplemental oxygen with a special oxygen regulator is required, as seen here. The photo is of Dr Clare O'Leary on the summit of Mount Everest in 2005. Courtesy of patfalvey.com.

Normal symptoms at altitude

- Hyperventilation (faster and deeper breathing) on exertion
- Periodic breathing
- Insomnia
- Increased urination
- Increased heart rate (up to 100 beats per minute)

Prevention is key!

Plan a gradual ascent that allows your body sufficient time to acclimatize. Be aware of the signs and symptoms of acute mountain sickness so you can identify and treat any problems early. It is important to remember that acclimatization occurs at different rates for different individuals. As a rule the following guidelines will prevent altitude illness in most individuals.

- Before going above 3000 m, spend at least one night at an intermediate elevation below 3000 m. It is not advisable to ascend from sea level up to above 3000 m without spending a night acclimatizing at approximately 2000 m. People do quite commonly fly into ski resorts from sea level and start skiing at 3000 m the following day. They should be made aware of the higher risk of developing acute mountain sickness

- Above 3000 m your sleeping elevation should not increase more than 300–500 m per night

- For every 1000 m gain in elevation you should spend a second night at the same elevation. When spending a second night at the same elevation it is useful to ascend to a higher elevation on a short trek during the intervening rest day, returning to the lower elevation to sleep. This helps acclimatization and allows recovery at night, ensuring you are ready for a longer ascent in the morning

Climb high, sleep low

- Avoid dehydration. Dehydration occurs more easily at altitude because of the increased breathing rate, which means that more moisture is lost from the lungs than normal

- Nutrition is important. On activity days a high carbohydrate diet is advised as carbohydrates require less oxygen to metabolize (burn) than fats and proteins, which should be eaten on rest days. Your energy requirements also increase to approximately 4000 kilocalories per day

- **Avoid** respiratory depressants (substances that reduce your drive to breathe):
  - Alcohol
  - Opioid painkillers
  - Sleeping tablets (at altitude do not treat insomnia with sleeping tablets – they will only exacerbate acute mountain sickness as they reduce your ability to breathe properly)

ALTITUDE ILLNESS

What should I check for?

Speak to the person

- When assessing a patient **the safety of both the rescuer and the patient is important.** For example, if on a glacier, **ensure everyone is attached to a safety rope**, then speak to the person

- Ensure the patient is conscious and can speak in complete sentences (see the ABC chapter (p. 21))

Problem identification – ask questions

- To assess if the person is orientated or confused
  - 'Where are you?'
  - 'What day and date is it?'
  - 'Who am I?'

- Confusion is a worrying sign and should be taken seriously

- Ask about other signs of acute mountain sickness:
  - 'Are you exhausted? Are you able to continue?'
  - 'Any nausea/vomiting?'
  - 'Any insomnia?'

Observe

- Is the person showing signs of exhaustion, e.g. slowing down or unable to continue?

- Is the person behaving inappropriately, e.g. undressing?

- Is there evidence that the person has difficulty breathing?

- Are their lips and extremities blue? Are they breathing rapidly at rest? Remember, being out of breath on exertion is normal as long the shortness of breath resolves with rest

- Is there evidence of dehydration, e.g. dry mucous

membranes, complaining of extreme thirst, confusion?

- Is the person walking in an unsteady manner as if drunk? Again, this is a worrying sign and should be taken seriously as it may indicate high altitude cerebral oedema (HACE) or high altitude pulmonary oedema (HAPE) **(Red Zone Conditions)** (see below)

Rule out serious injury

Assess for HACE and HAPE (see below). Both these conditions are potentially life-threatening and need immediate attention. If there is any suspicion of either of these conditions, immediate descent should begin. If symptoms do not improve on descent consider evacuation (e.g. air ambulance).

Touch

- If patient is unconscious start immediate assessment and management of ABCs (see the ABC chapter (p. 21))

- If oxygen and a delivery device are available oxygen should be applied at 4 litres/min

- Unfortunately, medical resources are often limited on remote mountain terrains where the majority of severe altitude illness presents

Skills assessment

- Is the person unable to keep up with the group?

- Assess how well the person can walk by asking them to heel–toe in a straight line. If staggering occurs, be suspicious of the presence of HACE

Denial of symptoms or attributing them to other minor illnesses is common, particularly on summit day when 'summit fever' takes over and climbers force themselves towards their goal. It's important to be alert to this and monitor closely anybody who is slowing down or unable to keep up. Unfortunately, some may progress to severe acute mountain illness before they make their symptoms known.

Acute mountain sickness

The spectrum of acute mountain illness ranges from mild acute mountain sickness to life-threatening HACE or HAPE. It occurs when your body fails to acclimatize or adapt to the lack of oxygen. At altitude everyone will develop hypoxia (decreased oxygen in the blood) to some extent. However, not everyone suffers from acute mountain sickness. Why some people tolerate hypoxia better than others is unknown. Acute mountain sickness typically occurs above 2500 m, with 75% of people experiencing symptoms above 3000 m. Mild acute mountain sickness is by far the most common form of altitude illness.

What should I check for?

A diagnosis of acute mountain illness is made when a **headache** with one or more of the following symptoms are present.

- **Gastrointestinal upset** – Is there any loss of appetite, nausea or vomiting?
- **Fatigue or weakness** – Is the person unable to keep up?
- **Dizziness** – Is the person complaining of dizziness or light-headedness?
- **Insomnia** – Is the person unable to sleep?

Other important questions that relate to the rate of ascent include

- At what elevation did the person sleep the previous night?
- Has the standard 300 m sleeping elevation gain per night been exceeded?
- How long have the symptoms been present?

A headache at altitude is never normal and should be assumed to be due to altitude illness until proven otherwise.

Dehydration is a common cause of non-acute-mountain-sickness headaches. The person should be given a litre of fluid to drink and a mild painkiller (aspirin or ibuprofen). If the headache does not resolve then the cause is more likely to be acute mountain sickness.

What should I do?

- **Rest** at minimum or descend – Stopping for rest is the minimum step in treating acute mountain sickness. If symptoms are severe immediate descent should be considered
- **Hydration** – Rehydrate with oral fluids
- **Painkillers** – Give paracetamol, aspirin or ibuprofen

The above three measures are usually adequate for most cases of acute mountain sickness. Once the person has recovered they may resume the ascent. If they remain symptomatic despite resting, or if features of HAPE or HACE develop, then **immediate descent is warranted**.

If in doubt, descend

Acetazolamide is a medication taken to prevent or treat acute mountain sickness. The recommended dose is 250 mg every 12 hours. For prophylaxis start taking acetazolamide at least 24 hours prior to ascending above 2500 m. It stimulates breathing and accelerates the acclimatization process. It does not mask symptoms. However it does not protect against worsening illness if ascending with symptoms. **It is not recommended to treat acute mountain illness by taking acetazolamide and continuing the ascent.**

High-altitude cerebral oedema

Altitude illness is a spectrum of illness ranging from mild symptoms as described above to life-threatening conditions such as HACE. This condition is due to swelling of brain tissue, which means the brain cannot work properly. The hallmark is an inability to think properly and an inability to coordinate movements. It is typically preceded by symptoms of acute mountain sickness which have been ignored or concealed.

What should I check for?

Patients with HACE will have **symptoms of acute mountain sickness** (see above) plus

- Unsteady walk (staggering as if drunk) – Ask the person to walk in a straight line heel–toe
- Mental status changes (confusion, disorientation) – Ask questions re time, day, date, place, etc.

Or just the above two signs together regardless of acute mountain sickness symptoms.

What should I do?

- **Descend immediately if possible** – HACE is a life-threatening condition. Untreated it can kill within hours. Immediate treatment involves ABC assessment (see the ABC chapter (p. 21)). **The need for descent is of the utmost urgency. Delay of even a few hours may have fatal consequences.** Descent should be at least 1000 m. The person will invariably need aid in the descent. They will need to be supported or even carried down. As medical resources are often limited, air ambulance evacuation (Fig. 20.4) may be required if symptoms do not improve
- **Consider medical treatments if available**

Medical treatments for high-altitude cerebral oedema

These treatments, where available, should ideally be administered by or in the presence of a qualified medical practitioner. There are used in the scenario **where descent/ evacuation is delayed** due to poor weather or the patient symptoms do not respond despite descending to a lower altitude. They are used as temporary measures to tide the person through until descent/ evacuation is possible.

- **Oxygen** – If oxygen is available it should be administered at 4 litres/ minute for 4–6 hours
- **Dexamethasone** – 8 mg intramuscularly immediately then 4 mg intramuscularly/ orally every 6 hours
- **Hyperbaric treatment** – This clever invention is an important device in treating HACE when it's available. It involves simulating descent by placing the individual in a sealed chamber (bag) and increasing the pressure within the bag by pumping air into it (Fig. 20.5). This has the effect of creating an atmosphere of lower altitude within the bag where the concentration of

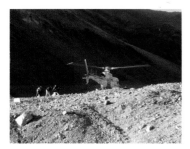

Fig. 20.4 Helicopter retrieval is sometimes necessary in cases of severe altitude illness.

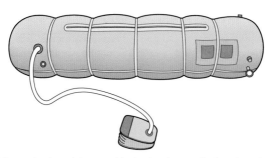

Fig. 20.5 A Gamow bag is an air-impermeable chamber that completely encloses the patient. The pressure is increased within the chamber by pumping air into it.

oxygen molecules has increased towards normal levels. Patients are treated in 1 hour segments, then re-evaluated. 4–6 hours is the optimal total treatment. These devices weigh approximately 6 kg and can be rented prior to a climbing trip

High-altitude pulmonary oedema

High-altitude pulmonary oedema is a severe form of altitude illness. It is not related to acute mountain sickness but it may occur alongside it. It causes a build-up of fluid in the lungs that leads to difficulty breathing. It usually occurs **during the night** after an ascent and is more frequent in younger climbers.

What should I check for?

Patients will have a combination of the following
- **Symptoms** – At least two of the following:
  - Breathless at rest
  - Cough
  - Severe fatigue or exercise intolerance
  - Chest tightness
- **Signs** – At least two of the following:
  - Wheezing

- Cyanosis (blue discoloration of lips)
- Fast pulse (>100 beats per minute)
- Rapid breathing

Severe fatigue or exercise intolerance is nearly always present, with an associated cough.

What should I do?

- If you are suspicious someone may have HAPE ask them to do a simple exercise test, e.g. ask them to walk 200 m and observe for above symptoms and signs
- **Descent as soon as possible to a medical unit is vital. Delay can result in death in a few hours. Even descent does not guarantee survival**
- Consider medical treatment if available

Medical treatment for high-altitude pulmonary oedema

These treatments, where available, should ideally be administered by or in the presence of a qualified medical practitioner.
- **Hyperbaric treatment** – As in HACE, the Gamow bag can give remarkable results if used early. One important difference is that the bag needs

to be tilted, as the patient will usually not tolerate lying flat. 2–4 hours is the optimal treatment time

- **Oxygen** is the most important treatment and should be administered at 4 litres/min for 4–6 hours

- **Nifedipine SR** – 20 mg four times daily orally – is a medication that can be given if available. It works by reducing the pressure in the blood vessels of the lungs allowing some of the fluid on the lungs to drain off

FINAL THOUGHTS

Altitude illness is now experienced by more people as

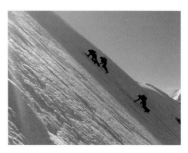

Fig. 20.6 On the ascent.

adventure travel gains in popularity. The key to avoiding altitude illness is to allow your body to acclimatize properly by ascending slowly, avoiding dehydration and eating a high-carbohydrate diet. If acute mountain illness develops the definitive cure is rapid descent.

After the Game

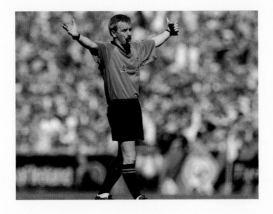

Player assessment

E Falvey, C McCarthy

Is the player OK?

- Any player injured during the game should be assessed after the match and referred for specialist review if there is any doubt. (Team Doctor/ Specialist)

Reassess/revisit the situation

- Be sure you know what actually happened and the nature of the player's complaint. This may be difficult in the heat of the moment during a game
- At times neither the player nor person attending them may be sure of the exact nature of the problem
- Having a chance to cool down and think about things can help both parties get to the bottom of the injury
- Simple indicators of seriousness of injury include:
  - Loss of full movement of the affected area

- Inability to weight bear
- Excess pain

Do: Use simple measures to promote a speedy recovery: PRICE

Protect
Make sure the affected area isn't hurt further.

Rest
Avoid further activity.

Ice
Regular icing will ease pain and reduce swelling. Care should be taken to avoid burning skin:

- Protect with a thin coating of oil/petroleum jelly
- Ice can be applied for 10–15 minutes every 2–3 hours

Elevate the affected area
Sit with foot on a pillow, arm in a sling.

- Foot above waist
- Wrist above elbow

Don't: HARM the area.

Heat
This can increase bleeding and swelling in an injury, worsening pain/stiffness.

Alcohol
This affects the player's ability to protect the injured area.

Running
Rest is the key to allow healing to occur.

Massage
In the early stage of an injury it is not of huge benefit and may cause harm.

Dehydration

- High intensity activity, particularly in hot or humid conditions, can lead to the loss of large amounts of fluid
- Players should drink before, during and after exercise
- The best way to ensure replacement of lost fluid is to weigh before and after the game, replacing lost weight with an equal amount of fluid
- Another useful guide is to monitor the appearance of urine produced; normally this should be clear and odourless
- With increasing dehydration, urine volume decreases, becomes more concentrated and appears darker

First aid

- Treat any minor abrasions/cut, etc, after a shower
- Clean affected area well with warm water
- Apply antiseptic spray/ ointment (e.g. Betadine, Savlon).

chapter 22

Event assessment

E Falvey, C McCarthy

INJURY AVOIDANCE

Could the injuries have been avoided by more comprehensive preparation?

Adequate protective equipment

- Is all playing equipment working properly and safely? Poorly maintained or ill-fitting playing equipment can jeopardize performance and directly result in injury

Was player size/experience/technique a factor?

- Players poorly matched for size and strength are prone to injury
- Those lacking experience need to be protected while they learn the necessary skills

Player fatigue

While fatigue is the natural result of playing/training with intensity, this should settle in 1–2 days, symptoms persisting longer need to be investigated. Excessive tiredness leads to training/playing errors and injury, as well as overuse injuries. The following factors can lead to excessive player fatigue:

- **Overtraining** – This can result from a coach unknowingly pushing an athlete beyond their ability, or an athlete, striving for better results, pushing harder than their body can tolerate. Conversely, this will lead to a drop in performance and is damaging both physically and mentally. A well-designed training programme with adequate rest/recovery periods is vital

- **Poor nutrition** – Inadequate calorific intake can affect performance and lead to injury. Players need to be advised on eating all the food groups regularly (protein, carbohydrate, fruit and vegetables, dairy products, nuts & cereals) – adequate protein intake is vital to maintain and grow hard-working muscle. Carbohydrate is essential to replace muscle energy stores

- **Inadequate sleep –** Players need adequate time in bed, at least 8 hours sleep is a minimum for those regularly active. Children and those involved in extremely strenuous exercise will require even more

Illness

As in the pre-match situation this must be monitored closely. Those obviously unwell do not present as much of a challenge as those who are 'borderline'. Looking at the players symptoms is vitally important.

- **Temperature –** No player with a temperature should train/play; instead, send them to their doctor

- Coughs and cold are common in winter time, a simple guide is **'the rule of the throat'** – if the player's symptoms are in the throat or above and they have no temperature they can be allowed to participate in light activities under observation. If this is tolerated with no ill effect then activity

may be increased. If the symptoms are below the throat, i.e. in their chest, they should be withheld from playing/training until such time as their symptoms have resolved. Attempting to play and train while ill will not only hamper performance but may lead to serious illness, e.g. myocarditis

Game preparation

Muscle tears may be avoided by a proper warm-up routine. Likewise, difficult training sessions in the days leading up to a game may cause muscle tightness and strain, predisposing the player to injury. Again, the importance of thoughtfully planning training to cater for players' weakness and prepare them for upcoming challenges cannot be stressed enough.

DEALING WITH THE INJURY

Was the injury recognized and coded appropriately (Red, Amber, Green)?

- Does this raise issues for the further management of injuries?

Was the injury managed properly?

* Was player injury dealt with in a timely and proper manner?

Detection of a struggling player and their removal from activity with quick implementation of treatment measures will prevent further injury and speed up the healing process. This must be our goal at all times. We mentioned earlier that 'a fit player is better than an injured star' – this must be borne in mind when a player, no matter how talented, begins to struggle with an injury.

When the player was removed from activity, was PRICE instituted and HARM avoided? Was medical/specialist opinion sought? A close working relationship with the physiotherapist or doctor looking after your team will ensure smooth passage of information in both directions. Always remember that the more those looking after an injury know about the injury

mechanism and the player they are treating, the better the outcome. Lessons can be learned from the injury circumstances and the rehabilitation implemented, to prevent further similar injury to the same player or others.

WHAT CAN WE DO TO IMPROVE CARE IN THE FUTURE?

As our players/athletes must train to improve their performance so must we constantly look at our performance and seek to improve it. By reading this book you are endeavouring to improve your ability to deal with potential adversity encountered by your players. This effort must be added to by ensuring that as many members of your organization as possible have first aid training. Contact your sports governing body for advice and assistance to help you improve your skills.

Index